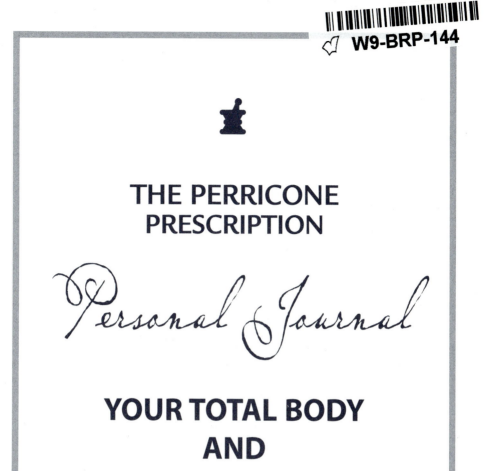

THE PERRICONE PRESCRIPTION

Personal Journal

YOUR TOTAL BODY
AND
FACE REJUVENATION
DAYBOOK

Nicholas Perricone, M.D.

HarperResource

An Imprint of HarperCollins *Publishers*

THE PERRICONE PRESCRIPTION PERSONAL JOURNAL. Copyright © 2002 by Nicholas Perricone, M.D. All rights reserved. Printed in the United States of America. No part of this book may be used or reproduced in any manner whatsoever without written permission except in the case of brief quotations embodied in critical articles and review. For information, address HarperCollins Publishers, Inc., 10 East 53rd Street, New York, NY 10022.

HarperCollins books may be purchased for educational, business, or sales promotional use. For information please write: Special Markets Department, HarperCollins Publishers, Inc., 10 East 53rd Street, New York, NY 10022.

FIRST EDITION
Designed by Lauren Steltzer

Library of Congress Cataloging-in-Publication Data
Perricone, Nicholas
    The Perricone prescription personal journal : your total body and face rejuvenation daybook / Nicholas Perricone.
        p. cm.
    ISBN 0-06-054161-X
        1. Skin—Care and hygiene. 2. Functional foods. 3. Dietary supplements. 4. Exercise—Health aspects. 5. Diaries—Authorship—Therapeutic use. I. Title.

RL87.P465 2002
613.7—dc21   2002032883

04 05 06   10   9 8 7 6 5 4

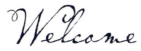

Welcome

I AM VERY PLEASED THAT YOU'VE TAKEN A SERIOUS INTEREST in the Perricone Prescription. I created this program for my patients, to help them understand and control the factors that affect their overall health and appearance. Understanding the "cause and effect" connection between daily activities (e.g., the foods we eat, the supplements we take, and the topical treatments we use) and physical well-being makes it simple to follow this scientifically-based program.

After working with thousands of patients over the fifteen years of my practice, I noticed that those who kept a *written* record of their progress tended to achieve better, more dramatic results. This journal has been specifically designed to complement my book *The Perricone Prescription*; recording your daily progress, as well as your thoughts and feelings as you make your way toward total body and face rejuvenation, will keep you focused and motivated.

This journal covers all aspects of my 28-Day Program. Each day's page outlines what you need to do from the moment you wake up until you go to bed at night. I provide your daily menus, the supplements you should take, and the skin care regimen you will follow. I outline a moderate exercise program and make recommendations for lifestyle changes, changes that will result in dramatic improvements in *all* aspects of your life. (A number of delicious recipes for meals included in the program—noted with an asterisk [*]—may be found in *The Perricone Prescription*, as are detailed exercise instructions and illustrations.)

Just as important as what I give you in this journal is what *you* contribute to it. That's why I ask for your written comments on your progress; each day you will record the changes you notice in your skin, your body, and your mood. This is a very important part of the program, and by keeping a record of your daily progress, you will find that your heightened sense of well-being—both physical and emotional—will further reinforce your commitment to this life-changing program.

On the next page I've provided spaces for "before" and "after" photos. Before you begin the Program, paste a recent photo of yourself in the "Day 1" space. Also note your body weight, as indicated. When you finish the first 28 days of the program, have a friend take another picture of you and paste that in the "Day 28" space. Don't forget to note your "after" weight, too. If you've followed my program faithfully, you should see dramatic results.

This journal has enough pages for three cycles of the 28-Day Program (roughly three months). Once you've completed three cycles, I'm confident that you'll choose to make the Perricone Program a permanent way of life.

Again, I'm very happy that you've decided to try the Perricone Prescription Program. I wish you well as you begin the enjoyable experience of attaining total body and face rejuvenation, and improve the quality of your life for years to come.

Sincerely,

Nicholas V. Perricone M.D

Nicholas Perricone, M.D.

DAY 1

"BEFORE" PHOTO

TOTAL BODY WEIGHT: _164_   1/1/06

DAY 28

"AFTER" PHOTO

TOTAL BODY WEIGHT: _____

Getting Started

THIS SECTION WILL TELL YOU EXACTLY WHAT YOU NEED to have on hand for the Perricone Prescription 28-Day Program—from food and supplements to skin care products and workout gear. Consult the Resource Section at the rear of this journal for recommended sources of some of the following selections.

✕

PHASE ONE PREPARATION: FOOD

Take a long, hard look at what you've got in your refrigerator and on your pantry shelves. Review the following lists and stock up on the nutritious, delicious foods that are recommended in my 28-day program.

Recommended protein:
Fish
- Albacore tuna
- Anchovies
- Bluefin tuna
- Halibut
- Herring
- Mackerel
- Sablefish

★Fish is the best all-around source of protein. The fish I recommend most highly is salmon, and I encourage you to eat salmon at least five times a week. However, the other cold-water fish I've listed may be used instead of salmon to add some variety to your diet.

- Salmon (Alaskan wild, not farm-raised)★
- Sardines
- Shad
- Shellfish
- Trout

Meat/Dairy
- Skinless and boneless chicken breast
- Turkey breast
- Turkey bacon
- Turkey sausage
- Eggs
- Plain whole milk yogurt
- Grating cheese (e.g., Parmesan, Romano)

> *If you are allergic to fish or are a strict vegetarian, your source of omega-3 essential fatty acids will be flax seed oil or fresh ground flax seed. Be sure to keep the oil and/or whole flax seeds refrigerated, as they are very fragile.*

Recommended vegetables:
- Arugula
- Asparagus
- Avocado
- Bean sprouts
- Broccoli and broccoli rabe
- Brussels sprouts
- Cauliflower
- Celery
- Cucumbers
- Eggplant
- Endive
- Escarole and other dark green leafy lettuces
- Garlic

- Ginger (fresh)
- Kale
- Mushrooms
- Onions (red and white)
- Peppers (green, orange, purple, red, and yellow)
- Romaine lettuce
- Spinach
- Summer squash
- Tomatoes
- Zucchini

Recommended fruits:
- Apples
- Berries (blackberries, blueberries, raspberries, and strawberries)
- Cantaloupe
- Cherries
- Honeydew melon
- Kiwi fruit
- Pears

Recommended beans and grains:
- Barley (whole, for soups)
- Beans (including black, chickpea, kidney, lentil, navy, pinto, and soy)
- Oatmeal (old-fashioned, coarse)

Recommended canned goods:
- Alaskan salmon
- Beans (black, chickpea, kidney, lentil, navy, pinto, and soy)
- Chicken broth (no-salt)
- Olives
- Sardines packed in olive oil
- Tuna

Recommended condiments:
- Extra virgin olive oil (Spanish olive oil is an excellent choice)

• Fresh lemon

Recommended snacks:

• Almonds
• Green and black olives
• Hazelnuts
• Macadamia nuts
• Walnuts
• 4 to 6 oz. whole milk yogurt mixed with 1 tsp. flax seed oil—
  a perfect snack of low-glycemic carbohydrates, protein, and
  essential fatty acids

Recommended beverages:

• Spring water
• Green or black tea

  Note: Iced green or black tea makes a refreshing, healthy
  beverage. Keep a pitcher in the refrigerator to enjoy throughout the day, served in a tall glass with a wedge of fresh lemon.

> **Protein First!**
> *Always remember to eat the protein first at* every *meal. It may
> seem odd to eat your fish before your soup, but doing so will
> ensure that you avoid a glycemic response.*

PHASE TWO PREPARATION: SUPPLEMENTS

Be sure to have an adequate supply of total skin and body supplements. These come pre-packaged in convenient individual
servings. (See the Resource Section for information on where to
find these supplements.)

• Take two supplement packets daily: one after breakfast, and
  one following lunch.

- Always take your supplements with a full glass of water (at least eight ounces).
- If taking the supplements in the morning causes stomach upset, take your first packet after lunch, and the second following dinner.

PHASE THREE PREPARATION: SKIN CARE

Clear your bathroom shelves and bureau top of harsh facial cleansers, scrubs, astringents, old creams, and expired sunscreen. Use recommended topicals as instructed below. (See the Resource Section for information on where to find these topical products.) For an extended list of recommended skin care products from various manufacturers, see *The Perricone Prescription*.

- Follow package insert instructions when beginning any new product. E.g., do a "patch test" first to ensure the product causes no irritation or allergic reaction.
- Topical products not included in the program should not be used in conjunction with recommended topicals, as irritation might result from the combination.
- Be very cautious if you are on prescription medication (topical or other) and/or undergoing facial acid peels, dermabrasion, or other aggressive dermatologic procedure, as irritation might result.

Following are the morning and evening skin care regimens recommended for the Perricone Prescription 28-Day Program.

Morning skin care
Cleanse: *Alpha Lipoic Acid Nutritive Cleanser*
Tone: *Alpha Lipoic Firming Facial Toner*
Treatment Face: *Alpha Lipoic Acid Face Firming Activator*

Treatment Eyes: *Alpha Lipoic Acid Eye Area Therapy; Vitamin C Ester Eye Area Therapy*
Treatment Lips: *Alpha Lipoic Acid Lip Plumper*
Moisturize Face and Neck (if needed): *Face Finishing Moisturizer*
Treatment Body: *Alpha Lipoic Acid Body Toning Lotion. (Use body toning lotion as needed throughout the day: after bath or shower; prior to sun exposure; to increase appearance of body tone, e.g., when wearing bathing suits, sleeveless shirts, shorts, etc.)*

Evening skin care
Repeat morning skin care; add Vitamin C Ester Concentrated Restorative Cream for face before bed.

PHASE FOUR PREPARATION: EXERCISE

Set aside at least twenty minutes each day for your aerobics or weight-training workout (remember to spend a few minutes warming up and cooling down). Pick a time of day that is convenient for you—we don't want your workout to become a source of stress! There's no guesswork involved, either; the type of exercise you should do each day is indicated in the program. Don't allow yourself to get in a rut—work out at a different time each day, whatever works best for your schedule. (While this program includes a daily workout, you may choose to exercise every other day rather than daily, depending on your fitness level. For example, if regular exercise is already a part of your life, you may not need to work out on a daily basis.)

The following gear is all you'll need to get a good daily workout:
• Comfortable, loose-fitting, "breathable" clothes
• Sturdy running shoes with good arch and ankle support
• Absorbent, cushioned socks

- A set of dumbbells and a set of ankle-weights. If you've never done weight-training before, begin using two-pound weights.
- An exercise mat (optional, but desired, especially as you increase your number of sit-ups)

It's not necessary to engage in rigorous and/or difficult physical activity to be fit; a daily twenty-minute walk provides tremendous health benefits, in addition to helping you de-stress and recharge. If you're just starting out, commit to a daily Perricone Prescription workout for at least 28 days—you'll soon look and feel so terrific that you'll be looking forward to your daily exercise!

PHASE FIVE PREPARATION: PERSONAL JOURNAL

As mentioned earlier, many of my patients find it helpful to keep a log to track their progress on the Perricone Program. Flip through the pages that follow to get a feel for the journal. There are two pages for each day. The left-hand page provides you with a step-by-step routine for the day: full food, supplement, topical, and exercise information. The right-hand page is to be used to note changes to your skin, body, and mind, and to record lifestyle activity. Use this page to examine your reactions and feelings, and to note more tangible results, e.g., weight, improvement in skin condition, increased energy. Whenever you feel tempted to stray from the program, take out your journal and jot down how you feel: did something happen to cause you to crave a specific food, want to skip your workout, or forgo your supplements? Becoming aware of the times, places, and feelings that induce you to stray from your goal will help you overcome temptation. Recording and bearing witness to your progress will inspire you to stick with it. (You'll notice that I've included space for "no-nos" – coffee, alcohol, and tobacco. Although these bad habits are *not* part of the Perricone Program, I encourage you to face up to them with honesty if they are a part of your life today so you may be free of them tomorrow.)

It is important to write in this journal every day. By focusing on and reviewing your day's activities, you will gain a greater appreciation of the physical and spiritual benefits that come from a healthy lifestyle. And there's nothing like measurable progress to keep you motivated to make the right choices for total health and good looks.

Finally, take the time to fill in the shaded box at the top of each day's right-hand page. Here I ask you to note three things that you appreciated that day. Some examples from my patients' journals include "watching a beautiful sunset," "running with my dog on the beach," and "sharing a laugh with my friends." This is a wonderful way to remind oneself of the joy and beauty that may be found every day of our lives.

Personal Journal

of

_____

WEEK 1 / DAY 1   DATE: _____

EXERCISE FOR THE DAY: *aerobics*

WAKE UP: *8-oz glass of water*

MORNING SKIN CARE

DIET

BREAKFAST
- 3 to 4 ounces smoked Nova Scotia salmon
- 1/2 cup slow-cooked oatmeal with 2 tablespoons blueberries
- 1 teaspoon slivered almonds
- Green or black tea or water
- 1 Total Skin & Body Vitamin Packet

LUNCH
- 4- to 6-ounce broiled turkey burger (no bun)
- Lettuce and tomato
- 1/2 cup Three-Bean Salad*
- Green or black tea or water
- 1 Total Skin & Body Vitamin Packet

AFTERNOON SNACK
- 2 ounces sliced turkey or chicken breast
- 4 hazelnuts
- 4 celery sticks
- Green or black tea or water

DINNER
- 4 to 6 ounces broiled salmon
- 1 cup lentil soup
- Tossed green salad dressed with olive oil and lemon juice
- 1/2 cup steamed spinach
- Green or black tea or water

BEDTIME SNACK
- 1 hard-boiled egg
- 3 celery sticks
- 3 red bell pepper strips
- 3 green olives

* Recipe available in *The Perricone Prescription: A Physician's 28-Day Program for Total Face and Body Rejuvenation.*

EVENING SKIN CARE

RECORD YOUR DAY'S ACTIVITIES, IMPRESSIONS, AND FEELINGS

TAKE A FEW MINUTES TO PRAY, MEDITATE, AND REFLECT

JOURNAL NOTES

THREE THINGS I APPRECIATED IN MY LIFE TODAY:

1. _____

2. _____

3. _____

SKIN

Face and Neck: _____   Fine Lines: _____

Dark Circles: _____   Puffiness: _____

Radiance: _____   Pore Size: _____

Firmness (jawline): _____

BODY

Weight: _____   Tone: _____

Energy: _____   Exercise: _____

MIND

Mood: _____   Stress: _____

Memory: _____   Problem-solving: _____

LIFESTYLE

Habits (coffee, alcohol, smoking): _____

Sleep (quality, number of hours): _____

Meditation/prayer: _____

OTHER NOTES, IMPRESSIONS, FEELINGS

_____

_____

_____

_____

WEEK 1 / DAY 2   DATE: _____

EXERCISE FOR THE DAY: *weight training*

WAKE UP: *8-oz glass of water*

 MORNING SKIN CARE

DIET

BREAKFAST
- Omelet made with 3 egg whites and one yolk
- Sliced tomato
- 1/2 cup blueberries
- Green or black tea or water
- 1 Total Skin & Body Vitamin Packet

LUNCH
- 3 to 6 ounces smoked or grilled salmon
- Green salad with tomatoes, cucumbers, onions and 2 tablespoons chickpeas dressed with olive oil, lemon juice, and garlic
- Green or black tea or water
- 1 Total Skin & Body Vitamin Packet

AFTERNOON SNACK
- 1/2 cup low-fat cottage cheese
- 4 small black olives
- 4 endive spears
- Green or black tea or water

DINNER
- 4 to 6 ounces baked or grilled halibut
- 1 cup Chicken-Vegetable Soup*
- Salad of romaine lettuce, chopped avocado, tomato, green onion, and celery dressed with olive oil and lemon juice
- Green or black tea or water

BEDTIME SNACK
- 2 ounces sliced roast turkey breast
- 6 whole almonds
- 3 red bell pepper strips
- 2-inch wedge of honeydew melon

* Recipe available in *The Perricone Prescription: A Physician's 28-Day Program for Total Face and Body Rejuvenation.*

EVENING SKIN CARE

RECORD YOUR DAY'S ACTIVITIES, IMPRESSIONS, AND FEELINGS

TAKE A FEW MINUTES TO PRAY, MEDITATE, AND REFLECT

JOURNAL NOTES

THREE THINGS I APPRECIATED IN MY LIFE TODAY:
1. _____
2. _____
3. _____

SKIN

Face and Neck: _____   Fine Lines: _____

Dark Circles: _____   Puffiness: _____

Radiance: _____   Pore Size: _____

Firmness (jawline): _____

BODY

Weight: _____   Tone: _____

Energy: _____   Exercise: _____

MIND

Mood: _____   Stress: _____

Memory: _____   Problem-solving: _____

LIFESTYLE

Habits (coffee, alcohol, smoking): _____

Sleep (quality, number of hours): _____

Meditation/prayer: _____

OTHER NOTES, IMPRESSIONS, FEELINGS

_____

_____

_____

_____

> *If you don't **drink water**, your body cannot metabolize fat.*

WEEK 1 / DAY 3   DATE: _____

 EXERCISE FOR THE DAY: *aerobics*

WAKE UP: *8-oz glass of water*

MORNING SKIN CARE

DIET

BREAKFAST
- 2 slices turkey bacon
- 6 ounces plain whole milk yogurt
- 1/2 cup strawberries
- Green or black tea or water
- 1 Total Skin & Body Vitamin Packet

LUNCH
- 3- to 4-ounce can water-packed tuna
- 1 cup sliced tomatoes and cucumbers
- 1/2 cup Three-Bean Salad*
- Green or black tea or water
- 1 Total Skin & Body Vitamin Packet

AFTERNOON SNACK
- 2 ounces sliced turkey breast
- 4 hazelnuts
- 1 small pear
- Green or black tea or water

DINNER
- 4 to 6 ounces broiled fillet of salmon. (Make 8 ounces and save
  2 ounces for tomorrow's bedtime snack.)
- 1/4 cup green beans
- Spinach salad with mushrooms, slice of red onion, and 1/4 cup
  chickpeas, dressed with olive oil and lemon juice
- Green or black tea or water

BEDTIME SNACK
- 2 ounces Grilled Chicken Breast*
- 1/4 cup raw cauliflower
- 4 black olives

* Recipe available in *The Perricone Prescription: A Physician's 28-Day Program for
Total Face and Body Rejuvenation.*

JOURNAL NOTES

THREE THINGS I APPRECIATED IN MY LIFE TODAY:

1. _____

2. _____

3. _____

SKIN

Face and Neck: _____   Fine Lines: _____

Dark Circles: _____   Puffiness: _____

Radiance: _____   Pore Size: _____

Firmness (jawline): _____

BODY

Weight: _____   Tone: _____

Energy: _____   Exercise: _____

MIND

Mood: _____   Stress: _____

Memory: _____   Problem-solving: _____

LIFESTYLE

Habits (coffee, alcohol, smoking): _____

Sleep (quality, number of hours): _____

Meditation/prayer: _____

OTHER NOTES, IMPRESSIONS, FEELINGS

_____

_____

_____

_____

> *Exercise in moderation has a **powerful, positive and anti-inflammatory** effect on our cells.*

WEEK 1 / DAY 4　　　DATE: _____

EXERCISE FOR THE DAY: *weight training*

WAKE UP: *8-oz glass of water*

MORNING SKIN CARE

DIET

BREAKFAST
- 1 slice of Canadian bacon or 2 slices turkey bacon
- 2 poached egg whites and one yolk
- $\frac{1}{2}$ cup slow-cooked oatmeal
- $\frac{1}{2}$ cup blueberries
- Green or black tea or water
- 1 Total Skin & Body Vitamin Packet

LUNCH
- 4 ounces grilled chicken salad (with fresh dill, chopped red onion, garlic, and olive oil)
- $\frac{1}{2}$ cup steamed broccoli
- $\frac{1}{2}$ cup strawberries
- Green or black tea or water
- 1 Total Skin & Body Vitamin Packet

AFTERNOON SNACK
- 2 slices roast turkey breast
- 4 cherry tomatoes
- 4 almonds
- Green or black tea or water

DINNER
- 6 ounces broiled fillet of sole, cod, or scrod.
- 8 Oven-Roasted Brussels Sprouts with Apples*
- Romaine lettuce salad with 2 ounces chickpeas, dressed with olive oil, garlic, and lemon juice
- Green or black tea or water

BEDTIME SNACK
- 2 ounces salmon
- 2 tablespoons Cuban Black Bean Salad*

* Recipe available in *The Perricone Prescription: A Physician's 28-Day Program for Total Face and Body Rejuvenation.*

EVENING SKIN CARE

RECORD YOUR DAY'S ACTIVITIES, IMPRESSIONS, AND FEELINGS

TAKE A FEW MINUTES TO PRAY, MEDITATE, AND REFLECT

JOURNAL NOTES

THREE THINGS I APPRECIATED IN MY LIFE TODAY:

1. _____

2. _____

3. _____

SKIN

Face and Neck: _____   Fine Lines: _____

Dark Circles: _____   Puffiness: _____

Radiance: _____   Pore Size: _____

Firmness (jawline): _____

BODY

Weight: _____   Tone: _____

Energy: _____   Exercise: _____

MIND

Mood: _____   Stress: _____

Memory: _____   Problem-solving: _____

LIFESTYLE

Habits (coffee, alcohol, smoking): _____

Sleep (quality, number of hours): _____

Meditation/prayer: _____

OTHER NOTES, IMPRESSIONS, FEELINGS

_____

_____

_____

_____

> *Salmon for breakfast greatly facilitates **weight loss
> and appetite control.***

Week 1 / Day 5   Date: _____

✚ **Exercise for the day:** *aerobics (20 minutes' vigorous walking)*

💧 **Wake up:** *8-oz glass of water*

🧴 **Morning skin care**

✗ **Diet**

BREAKFAST
- 4 ounces smoked salmon
- $^1/_2$ cup slow-cooked oatmeal seasoned with cinnamon
- 2 teaspoons chopped almonds
- 2-inch wedge of cantaloupe
- Green or black tea or water
- 1 Total Skin & Body Vitamin Packet

LUNCH
- 4 ounces salmon salad (finely cubed salmon fillet or canned salmon dressed with lemon juice, olive oil, and dill) served on a bed of romaine lettuce
- $^1/_2$ cup lentil soup
- Green or black tea or water
- 1 Total Skin & Body Vitamin Packet

AFTERNOON SNACK
- 2 slices turkey breast
- $^1/_2$ cup strawberries
- 4 hazelnuts
- Green or black tea or water

DINNER
- 1 roast chicken breast (skin removed)
- $^1/_2$ cup grilled zucchini
- $^1/_2$ cup Three Bean Salad*
- Green or black tea or water

BEDTIME SNACK
- 2 ounces drained canned shrimp or tuna
- 3 macadamia nuts
- 3 cherry tomatoes

* Recipe available in *The Perricone Prescription: A Physician's 28-Day Program for Total Face and Body Rejuvenation.*

- **EVENING SKIN CARE**
- **RECORD YOUR DAY'S ACTIVITIES, IMPRESSIONS, AND FEELINGS**
- **TAKE A FEW MINUTES TO PRAY, MEDITATE, AND REFLECT**

JOURNAL NOTES

THREE THINGS I APPRECIATED IN MY LIFE TODAY:

1. _____
2. _____
3. _____

SKIN

Face and Neck: _____   Fine Lines: _____

Dark Circles: _____   Puffiness: _____

Radiance: _____   Pore Size: _____

Firmness (jawline): _____

BODY

Weight: _____   Tone: _____

Energy: _____   Exercise: _____

MIND

Mood: _____   Stress: _____

Memory: _____   Problem-solving: _____

LIFESTYLE

Habits (coffee, alcohol, smoking): _____

Sleep (quality, number of hours): _____

Meditation/prayer: _____

OTHER NOTES, IMPRESSIONS, FEELINGS

_____

_____

_____

_____

> *Not all fats are bad—and **the right fats** can help you lose weight.*

WEEK 1 / DAY 6   DATE: _____

 EXERCISE FOR THE DAY: *weight training*

WAKE UP: *8-oz glass of water*

MORNING SKIN CARE

DIET

BREAKFAST
- Omelet of 3 egg whites and 1 yolk with a few sliced mushrooms and $^1/_2$ cup chopped spinach
- 1 slice Canadian or turkey bacon
- 2-inch wedge of honeydew melon
- Green or black tea or water
- 1 Total Skin & Body Vitamin Packet

LUNCH
- 4 to 6 ounces broiled salmon
- Caesar salad without croutons
- $^1/_2$ apple
- Green or black tea or water
- 1 Total Skin & Body Vitamin Packet

AFTERNOON SNACK
- 1 hard-boiled egg
- $^1/_2$ cup sliced strawberries
- 3 almonds
- Green or black tea or water

DINNER
- 4 to 6 ounces grilled halibut
- Tossed Greek salad made with romaine lettuce, 3 black olives, 1 ounce feta cheese, $^1/_2$ cucumber, 4 cherry tomatoes; dressed with olive oil, lemon juice, and a dash of oregano, mixed to taste
- Steamed or Grilled Asparagus*
- 2-inch wedge of cataloupe
- Green or black tea or water

BEDTIME SNACK
- 2 slices roast turkey or chicken breast
- 4 macadamia nuts
- Small peach or nectarine

* Recipe available in *The Perricone Prescription: A Physician's 28-Day Program for Total Face and Body Rejuvenation.*

EVENING SKIN CARE

RECORD YOUR DAY'S ACTIVITIES, IMPRESSIONS, AND FEELINGS

TAKE A FEW MINUTES TO PRAY, MEDITATE, AND REFLECT

JOURNAL NOTES

THREE THINGS I APPRECIATED IN MY LIFE TODAY:

1. _____
2. _____
3. _____

SKIN

Face and Neck: _____   Fine Lines: _____

Dark Circles: _____   Puffiness: _____

Radiance: _____   Pore Size: _____

Firmness (jawline): _____

BODY

Weight: _____   Tone: _____

Energy: _____   Exercise: _____

MIND

Mood: _____   Stress: _____

Memory: _____   Problem-solving: _____

LIFESTYLE

Habits (coffee, alcohol, smoking): _____

Sleep (quality, number of hours): _____

Meditation/prayer: _____

OTHER NOTES, IMPRESSIONS, FEELINGS

_____

_____

_____

_____

> *A diet rich in **extra virgin olive oil** increases the skin's ability to maintain moisture, lowers blood pressure, prevents osteoporosis, reduces the risk of certain cancers...*
> *and much more.*

WEEK 1 / DAY 7   DATE: _____

EXERCISE FOR THE DAY: *relaxation (you've earned it!)*

WAKE UP: *8-oz glass of water*

MORNING SKIN CARE

DIET

BREAKFAST
· 3 to 6 ounces broiled salmon
· $^1/_2$ cup slow-cooked oatmeal
· 2-inch wedge of cantaloupe
· Green or black tea or water
· 1 Total Skin & Body Vitamin Packet

LUNCH
· Crabmeat salad made with a 6-ounce can of crabmeat, 1 chopped scallion, 1 chopped celery rib; dress with $^1/_4$ cup yogurt, juice of $^1/_2$ lemon; serve inside $^1/_2$ avocado
· 1 cup strawberries
· Green or black tea or water
· 1 Total Skin & Body Vitamin Packet

AFTERNOON SNACK
· $^1/_2$ cup cottage cheese
· 4 almonds
· 1 apple
· Green or black tea or water

DINNER
· Grilled chicken breast*
· $^3/_4$ cup roasted or sautéed mushrooms and Sautéed Zucchini or Summer Squash*
· Romaine lettuce salad, sliced tomatoes, fresh basil with 1 ounce grated Parmesan cheese, dressed with olive oil and lemon juice, mixed to taste
· Green or black tea or water

BEDTIME SNACK
· 2 slices of turkey breast
· 3 olives
· 1 pear

* Recipe available in *The Perricone Prescription: A Physician's 28-Day Program for Total Face and Body Rejuvenation.*

◻️ EVENING SKIN CARE

📖 RECORD YOUR DAY'S ACTIVITIES, IMPRESSIONS, AND FEELINGS

☁️ TAKE A FEW MINUTES TO PRAY, MEDITATE, AND REFLECT

JOURNAL NOTES

THREE THINGS I APPRECIATED IN MY LIFE TODAY:
1. _____
2. _____
3. _____

SKIN

Face and Neck: _____   Fine Lines: _____

Dark Circles: _____   Puffiness: _____

Radiance: _____   Pore Size: _____

Firmness (jawline): _____

BODY

Weight: _____   Tone: _____

Energy: _____   Exercise: _____

MIND

Mood: _____   Stress: _____

Memory: _____   Problem-solving: _____

LIFESTYLE

Habits (coffee, alcohol, smoking): _____

Sleep (quality, number of hours): _____

Meditation/prayer: _____

OTHER NOTES, IMPRESSIONS, FEELINGS

_____

_____

_____

_____

> *Alpha lipoic acid is a **natural substance** found in our bodies—and it is one of the most powerful anti-aging, antioxidant, anti-inflammatories available.*

WEEK 2 / DAY 8   DATE: _____

EXERCISE FOR THE DAY: *aerobics (20 minutes' vigorous walking)*

WAKE UP: *8-oz glass of water*

MORNING SKIN CARE

DIET

BREAKFAST
- 2 slices Canadian bacon, ham, or turkey bacon
- 1/2 cup plain cottage cheese
- 1/2 cup blueberries
- Green or black tea or water
- 1 Total Skin & Body Vitamin Packet

LUNCH
- 3- to 4-ounce can water-packed tuna
- 1/2 cup lentil soup
- Romaine lettuce salad topped with chopped tomato and red onion; dress with olive oil and lemon
- Green or black tea or water
- 1 Total Skin & Body Vitamin Packet

AFTERNOON SNACK
- 2 ounces smoked salmon
- 3 hazelnuts
- 2-inch wedge cantaloupe
- Green or black tea or water

DINNER
- 6 ounces Scallops with Garlic and Parsley* (cook 8 ounces and save 2 ounces for tomorrow's lunch)
- Mediterranean Chopped Salad* with 1/2 cup chickpeas
- 1/2 cup cooked green beans
- Green or black tea or water

BEDTIME SNACK
- 2 slices turkey breast
- 4 green olives
- 1 apple

* Recipe available in *The Perricone Prescription: A Physician's 28-Day Program for Total Face and Body Rejuvenation.*

EVENING SKIN CARE

RECORD YOUR DAY'S ACTIVITIES, IMPRESSIONS, AND FEELINGS

TAKE A FEW MINUTES TO PRAY, MEDITATE, AND REFLECT

JOURNAL NOTES

THREE THINGS I APPRECIATED IN MY LIFE TODAY:
1. _____
2. _____
3. _____

SKIN

Face and Neck: _____   Fine Lines: _____

Dark Circles: _____   Puffiness: _____

Radiance: _____   Pore Size: _____

Firmness (jawline): _____

BODY

Weight: _____   Tone: _____

Energy: _____   Exercise: _____

MIND

Mood: _____   Stress: _____

Memory: _____   Problem-solving: _____

LIFESTYLE

Habits (coffee, alcohol, smoking): _____

Sleep (quality, number of hours): _____

Meditation/prayer: _____

OTHER NOTES, IMPRESSIONS, FEELINGS

_____

_____

_____

_____

WEEK 2 / DAY 9   **DATE:** _____

 EXERCISE FOR THE DAY: *weight training*

WAKE UP: *8-oz glass of water*

MORNING SKIN CARE

DIET

BREAKFAST
- Egg white omelet made with 3 to 4 egg whites and one yolk (add a few sliced mushrooms, if desired)
- 1/2 cup slow-cooked oatmeal
- 3 hazelnuts
- Green or black tea or water
- 1 Total Skin & Body Vitamin Packet

LUNCH
- Scallop salad (2 ounces scallops from previous night's dinner); dressed with olive oil, lemon juice, chopped red onion, and dill
- 1/2 cup Three Bean Salad*
- Green or black tea or water
- 1 Total Skin & Body Vitamin Packet

AFTERNOON SNACK
- 2 ounces smoked salmon
- 4 black olives
- 3 endive spears
- Green or black tea or water

DINNER
- 6 ounces grilled salmon
- 1/2 cup Cuban Black Bean Soup*
- Romaine salad dressed with olive oil and lemon juice
- 1/2 cup berries
- Green or black tea or water

BEDTIME SNACK
- 6 ounces plain whole milk yogurt or cottage cheese
- 1/2 cup strawberries
- 4 macadamia nuts

* Recipe available in *The Perricone Prescription: A Physician's 28-Day Program for Total Face and Body Rejuvenation.*

JOURNAL NOTES

THREE THINGS I APPRECIATED IN MY LIFE TODAY:

1. _____
2. _____
3. _____

SKIN

Face and Neck: _____ Fine Lines: _____

Dark Circles: _____ Puffiness: _____

Radiance: _____ Pore Size: _____

Firmness (jawline): _____

BODY

Weight: _____ Tone: _____

Energy: _____ Exercise: _____

MIND

Mood: _____ Stress: _____

Memory: _____ Problem-solving: _____

LIFESTYLE

Habits (coffee, alcohol, smoking): _____

Sleep (quality, number of hours): _____

Meditation/prayer: _____

OTHER NOTES, IMPRESSIONS, FEELINGS

_____

_____

_____

_____

> **Be kind to your face** and it will be kind to you. Use a
> gentle liquid cleanser applied by hand, then rinsed off
> thoroughly with lukewarm water.

WEEK 2 / DAY 10   DATE: _____

 EXERCISE FOR THE DAY: *aerobics*

WAKE UP: *8-oz glass of water*

MORNING SKIN CARE

DIET

BREAKFAST
· 2 slices turkey bacon
· 1 cup plain whole milk yogurt
· 1/2 cup strawberries
· 3 almonds
· Green or black tea or water
· 1 Total Skin & Body Vitamin Packet

LUNCH
· 4 to 6 ounces grilled chicken
· 1/2 cup vegetable barley soup
· Large green salad with sliced tomatoes
· 2-inch wedge of cantaloupe
· Green or black tea or water
· 1 Total Skin & Body Vitamin Packet

AFTERNOON SNACK
· 1 hard-boiled egg
· 2-inch wedge of cantaloupe
· 4 almonds
· Green or black tea or water

DINNER
· 6 ounces Scallops with Garlic and Parsley*
· Mediterranean Chopped Salad* with 1/2 cup chickpeas
· 1/2 cup cooked green beans
· Green or black tea or water

BEDTIME SNACK
· 2 slices turkey breast
· 4 green olives
· 1 apple

* Recipe available in *The Perricone Prescription: A Physician's 28-Day Program for
Total Face and Body Rejuvenation.*

EVENING SKIN CARE

RECORD YOUR DAY'S ACTIVITIES, IMPRESSIONS, AND FEELINGS

TAKE A FEW MINUTES TO PRAY, MEDITATE, AND REFLECT

JOURNAL NOTES

THREE THINGS I APPRECIATED IN MY LIFE TODAY:

1. _____

2. _____

3. _____

SKIN

Face and Neck: _____   Fine Lines: _____

Dark Circles: _____   Puffiness: _____

Radiance: _____   Pore Size: _____

Firmness (jawline): _____

BODY

Weight: _____   Tone: _____

Energy: _____   Exercise: _____

MIND

Mood: _____   Stress: _____

Memory: _____   Problem-solving: _____

LIFESTYLE

Habits (coffee, alcohol, smoking): _____

Sleep (quality, number of hours): _____

Meditation/prayer: _____

OTHER NOTES, IMPRESSIONS, FEELINGS

_____

_____

_____

_____

WEEK 2 / DAY 11 DATE: _____

 EXERCISE FOR THE DAY: *weight training*

WAKE UP: *8-oz glass of water*

MORNING SKIN CARE

DIET

BREAKFAST
- 4 ounces smoked salmon
- 3 ounces plain whole milk yogurt
- 1 tomato slice
- 1/4 cantaloupe
- Green or black tea or water
- 1 Total Skin & Body Vitamin Packet

LUNCH
- 6 ounces canned crabmeat dressed with 1 tablespoon mayonnaise
- 1/2 cup lentil soup
- Large romaine lettuce salad dressed with olive oil and lemon to taste
- Green or black tea or water
- 1 Total Skin & Body Vitamin Packet

AFTERNOON SNACK
- 1 hard-boiled egg
- 4 cherry tomatoes
- 4 macadamia nuts
- Green or black tea or water

DINNER
- 6 ounces roast chicken breast (cook 8 ounces and save 2 ounces for tomorrow's lunch)
- 1/2 cup Manhattan Clam Chowder*
- 1/2 cup grilled eggplant topped with sliced tomato and 1 tablespoon grated Parmesan cheese
- Green or black tea or water

BEDTIME SNACK
- 1/2 cup cottage cheese
- 1/2 cup blueberries
- 4 hazelnuts

* Recipe available in *The Perricone Prescription: A Physician's 28-Day Program for Total Face and Body Rejuvenation.*

■ Evening skin care

□ Record your day's activities, impressions, and feelings

☁ Take a few minutes to pray, meditate, and reflect

Journal Notes

THREE THINGS I APPRECIATED IN MY LIFE TODAY:

1. _____

2. _____

3. _____

SKIN

Face and Neck: _____   Fine Lines: _____

Dark Circles: _____   Puffiness: _____

Radiance: _____   Pore Size: _____

Firmness (jawline): _____

BODY

Weight: _____   Tone: _____

Energy: _____   Exercise: _____

MIND

Mood: _____   Stress: _____

Memory: _____   Problem-solving: _____

LIFESTYLE

Habits (coffee, alcohol, smoking): _____

Sleep (quality, number of hours): _____

Meditation/prayer: _____

OTHER NOTES, IMPRESSIONS, FEELINGS

_____

_____

_____

_____

> *An ongoing lack of protein is always **noticeable**
> in the face first.*

WEEK 2 / DAY 12 DATE: _____

 EXERCISE FOR THE DAY: *aerobics (20 minutes' vigorous walking)*

WAKE UP: *8-oz glass of water*

MORNING SKIN CARE

DIET

BREAKFAST
· Scrambled eggs (3 egg whites and 1 yolk) with a little chopped onion
  and green bell peppers
· 2 slices turkey bacon
· 2-inch wedge cantaloupe
· Green or black tea or water
· 1 Total Skin & Body Vitamin Packet

LUNCH
· 3 to 5 ounces of chicken salad (made with 2 ounces chicken saved
  from last night's dinner, mixed with chopped red onion and celery,
  and dressed with 1 tablespoon olive oil and lemon juice) served on
  a bed of romaine lettuce
· Sliced tomatoes
· 1 cup Chicken-Vegetable Soup*
· Green or black tea or water
· 1 Total Skin & Body Vitamin Packet

AFTERNOON SNACK
· ½ cup plain whole milk yogurt
· ½ cup blueberries
· 1 teaspoon chopped almonds
· Green or black tea or water

DINNER
· 6 ounces grilled salmon
· Salad of romaine lettuce, avocado, and tomato, dressed with olive oil
  and lemon juice
· Grilled zucchini and mushroom kebabs
· Green or black tea or water

BEDTIME SNACK
· 2 ounces tuna salad (tuna mixed with onion, celery, pepper, and
  mustard or a touch or mayonnaise, if desired)
· 4 almonds
· 1 pear

* Recipe available in *The Perricone Prescription: A Physician's 28-Day Program for
Total Face and Body Rejuvenation.*

EVENING SKIN CARE

RECORD YOUR DAY'S ACTIVITIES, IMPRESSIONS, AND FEELINGS

TAKE A FEW MINUTES TO PRAY, MEDITATE, AND REFLECT

JOURNAL NOTES

THREE THINGS I APPRECIATED IN MY LIFE TODAY:

1. _____
2. _____
3. _____

SKIN

Face and Neck: _____ Fine Lines: _____

Dark Circles: _____ Puffiness: _____

Radiance: _____ Pore Size: _____

Firmness (jawline): _____

BODY

Weight: _____ Tone: _____

Energy: _____ Exercise: _____

MIND

Mood: _____ Stress: _____

Memory: _____ Problem-solving: _____

LIFESTYLE

Habits (coffee, alcohol, smoking): _____

Sleep (quality, number of hours): _____

Meditation/prayer: _____

OTHER NOTES, IMPRESSIONS, FEELINGS

_____

_____

_____

_____

> *Olive oil is one of **nature's greatest gifts** for preserving your health, beauty, and longevity.*

WEEK 2 / DAY 13   DATE: _____

 EXERCISE FOR THE DAY: *aerobics*

WAKE UP: *8-oz glass of water*

MORNING SKIN CARE

DIET

BREAKFAST
- 2 to 4 ounces smoked salmon
- 1/2 cup plain whole milk yogurt
- 1 tablespoon chopped walnuts
- 1/2 cup blueberries
- Green or black tea or water
- 1 Total Skin & Body Vitamin Packet

LUNCH
- Grilled Chicken Breast*
- Green salad topped with 1/2 cup white or navy beans
- Steamed asparagus
- Green or black tea or water
- 1 Total Skin & Body Vitamin Packet

AFTERNOON SNACK
- 1 hard-boiled egg
- 2-inch wedge cantaloupe
- 4 macadamia nuts
- Green or black tea or water

DINNER
- 6 ounces grilled bluefin or albacore tuna steak
- 1/2 cup grilled zucchini, eggplant, and red or green bell peppers lightly drizzled with olive oil and sprinkled with 1 tablespoon Parmesan cheese
- Tomato salsa (use fresh, if possible)
- Green or black tea or water

BEDTIME SNACK
- 2 slices turkey breast
- 4 green olives
- 4 cherry tomatoes

* Recipe available in *The Perricone Prescription: A Physician's 28-Day Program for Total Face and Body Rejuvenation.*

JOURNAL NOTES

THREE THINGS I APPRECIATED IN MY LIFE TODAY:
1. _____
2. _____
3. _____

SKIN

Face and Neck: _____   Fine Lines: _____

Dark Circles: _____   Puffiness: _____

Radiance: _____   Pore Size: _____

Firmness (jawline): _____

BODY

Weight: _____   Tone: _____

Energy: _____   Exercise: _____

MIND

Mood: _____   Stress: _____

Memory: _____   Problem-solving: _____

LIFESTYLE

Habits (coffee, alcohol, smoking): _____

Sleep (quality, number of hours): _____

Meditation/prayer: _____

OTHER NOTES, IMPRESSIONS, FEELINGS

_____

_____

_____

_____

> *A dehydrated body provokes the development of aging. Even mild dehydration can result in the gain of* **one pound of fat every six months.**

WEEK 2 / DAY 14   DATE: _____

✛ EXERCISE FOR THE DAY: *relaxation (you've* **REALLY** *earned it!)*

💧 WAKE UP: *8-oz glass of water*

🧴 MORNING SKIN CARE

✗ DIET

BREAKFAST
· Omelet made with 3 egg whites, 1 yolk, and a few sliced fresh mushrooms
· $1/2$ cup slow-cooked oatmeal
· 1 teaspoon chopped almonds
· 2-inch wedge cantaloupe
· Green or black tea or water
· 1 Total Skin & Body Vitamin Packet

LUNCH
· 3 to 4 ounces water-packed tuna
· Romaine lettuce salad made with $1/2$ cup white beans, $1/4$ cup crumbled feta cheese, 4 cherry tomatoes, and sliced red onion, dressed with olive oil and lemon juice
· Green or black tea or water
· 1 Total Skin & Body Vitamin Packet

AFTERNOON SNACK
· 1 slice turkey breast
· 4 hazelnuts
· 2-inch wedge cantaloupe
· Green or black tea or water

DINNER
· 4 large shrimp, grilled, broiled, or baked on skewers with mushrooms, onions, and cherry tomatoes
· $1/2$ cup Cuban Black Bean Soup*
· Romaine lettuce salad dressed with olive oil and lemon juice
· Green or black tea or water

BEDTIME SNACK
· 2 slices turkey breast
· 4 green olives
· 4 cherry tomatoes

* Recipe available in *The Perricone Prescription: A Physician's 28-Day Program for Total Face and Body Rejuvenation.*

EVENING SKIN CARE

RECORD YOUR DAY'S ACTIVITIES, IMPRESSIONS, AND FEELINGS

TAKE A FEW MINUTES TO PRAY, MEDITATE, AND REFLECT

JOURNAL NOTES

THREE THINGS I APPRECIATED IN MY LIFE TODAY:
1. _____
2. _____
3. _____

SKIN

Face and Neck: _____   Fine Lines: _____

Dark Circles: _____   Puffiness: _____

Radiance: _____   Pore Size: _____

Firmness (jawline): _____

BODY

Weight: _____   Tone: _____

Energy: _____   Exercise: _____

MIND

Mood: _____   Stress: _____

Memory: _____   Problem-solving: _____

LIFESTYLE

Habits (coffee, alcohol, smoking): _____

Sleep (quality, number of hours): _____

Meditation/prayer: _____

OTHER NOTES, IMPRESSIONS, FEELINGS

_____
_____
_____
_____

> *Drinking hard liquor causes inflammatory problems in the body. In short: wine is fine… but **forget the martini**.*

WEEK 3 / DAY 15   DATE: _____

EXERCISE FOR THE DAY: *aerobics (20 minutes' vigorous walking)*

WAKE UP: *8-oz glass of water*

MORNING SKIN CARE

DIET

BREAKFAST
- 2 ounces smoked salmon
- 6 ounces plain whole milk yogurt
- 2-inch wedge cantaloupe
- Green or black tea or water
- 1 Total Skin & Body Vitamin Packet

LUNCH
- 1 6-ounce can shrimp (drained) mixed with 1 tablespoon olive oil and juice of $1/2$ lemon, served inside $1/2$ avocado
- $1/2$ cup cherries
- Green or black tea or water
- 1 Total Skin & Body Vitamin Packet

AFTERNOON SNACK
- 2 ounces sliced turkey or chicken breast
- 4 almonds
- 4 cherry tomatoes
- Green or black tea or water

DINNER
- 4 to 6 ounces baked scrod fillets
- $1/2$ cup steamed broccoli or spinach
- Tossed green salad dressed with olive oil and lemon juice
- Green or black tea or water

BEDTIME SNACK
- 1 hard-boiled egg
- 3 celery sticks
- 3 green olives

EVENING SKIN CARE

RECORD YOUR DAY'S ACTIVITIES, IMPRESSIONS, AND FEELINGS

TAKE A FEW MINUTES TO PRAY, MEDITATE, AND REFLECT

JOURNAL NOTES

THREE THINGS I APPRECIATED IN MY LIFE TODAY:

1. _____

2. _____

3. _____

SKIN

Face and Neck: _____   Fine Lines: _____

Dark Circles: _____   Puffiness: _____

Radiance: _____   Pore Size: _____

Firmness (jawline): _____

BODY

Weight: _____   Tone: _____

Energy: _____   Exercise: _____

MIND

Mood: _____   Stress: _____

Memory: _____   Problem-solving: _____

LIFESTYLE

Habits (coffee, alcohol, smoking): _____

Sleep (quality, number of hours): _____

Meditation/prayer: _____

OTHER NOTES, IMPRESSIONS, FEELINGS

_____

_____

_____

_____

> *A **good night's sleep** can help you awake refreshed, looking radiant and youthful. And, after a good night's sleep, doesn't the world look better, too?*

WEEK 3 / DAY 16   DATE: _____

EXERCISE FOR THE DAY: *weight training*

WAKE UP: *8-oz glass of water*

MORNING SKIN CARE

DIET

BREAKFAST
- Omelet made with 2 eggs, fresh herbs, and a few sliced fresh mushrooms
- $1/2$ cup slow-cooked oatmeal
- 3 hazelnuts
- $1/2$ cup blueberries
- Green or black tea or water
- 1 Total Skin & Body Vitamin Packet

LUNCH
- 3 to 6 ounces canned salmon mixed with 1 teaspoon mayonnaise
- Green salad with sliced tomatoes, cucumbers, and 2 tablespoons chickpeas; dressed with olive oil and lemon juice
- 2-inch wedge honeydew melon
- Green or black tea or water
- 1 Total Skin & Body Vitamin Packet

AFTERNOON SNACK
- 6 ounces plain whole milk yogurt
- 3 hazelnuts
- $1/4$ cup fresh berries
- Green or black tea or water

DINNER
- 4 to 6 ounces baked or grilled trout
- $1/2$ cup Three-Bean Salad*
- $1/2$ cup steamed and mashed turnip
- 1 pear
- Green or black tea or water

BEDTIME SNACK
- 2 ounces sliced roast turkey breast
- 4 almonds
- 3 radishes

* Recipe available in *The Perricone Prescription: A Physician's 28-Day Program for Total Face and Body Rejuvenation.*

JOURNAL NOTES

THREE THINGS I APPRECIATED IN MY LIFE TODAY:

1. _____
2. _____
3. _____

SKIN

Face and Neck: _____   Fine Lines: _____

Dark Circles: _____   Puffiness: _____

Radiance: _____   Pore Size: _____

Firmness (jawline): _____

BODY

Weight: _____   Tone: _____

Energy: _____   Exercise: _____

MIND

Mood: _____   Stress: _____

Memory: _____   Problem-solving: _____

LIFESTYLE

Habits (coffee, alcohol, smoking): _____

Sleep (quality, number of hours): _____

Meditation/prayer: _____

OTHER NOTES, IMPRESSIONS, FEELINGS

_____
_____
_____
_____

WEEK 3 / DAY 17   DATE: _____

 EXERCISE FOR THE DAY: *aerobics*

WAKE UP: *8-oz glass of water*

MORNING SKIN CARE

DIET

BREAKFAST
- 2 slices turkey bacon
- 1/2 cup slow-cooked oatmeal
- 3 hazelnuts
- 1/2 grapefruit
- Green or black tea or water
- 1 Total Skin & Body Vitamin Packet

LUNCH
- 3- to 4-ounce can tuna or sardines
- 1 cup sliced tomatoes and cucumbers
- 1/2 cup lentil soup
- Green or black tea or water
- 1 Total Skin & Body Vitamin Packet

AFTERNOON SNACK
- 6 ounces plain whole milk yogurt
- 4 chopped almonds
- 1 small apple
- Green or black tea or water

DINNER
- 4 to 6 ounces broiled fillet of salmon (make 8 ounces and save 2 ounces for tomorrow's bedtime snack)
- 1 cup steamed asparagus
- Romaine lettuce salad with 1/4 cup chickpeas; dressed with olive oil and lemon juice
- Green or black tea or water

BEDTIME SNACK
- 2 ounces sliced turkey or chicken breast
- 4 black olives
- 1 kiwi fruit

EVENING SKIN CARE

RECORD YOUR DAY'S ACTIVITIES, IMPRESSIONS, AND FEELINGS

TAKE A FEW MINUTES TO PRAY, MEDITATE, AND REFLECT

JOURNAL NOTES

THREE THINGS I APPRECIATED IN MY LIFE TODAY:

1. _____
2. _____
3. _____

SKIN

Face and Neck: _____ Fine Lines: _____

Dark Circles: _____ Puffiness: _____

Radiance: _____ Pore Size: _____

Firmness (jawline): _____

BODY

Weight: _____ Tone: _____

Energy: _____ Exercise: _____

MIND

Mood: _____ Stress: _____

Memory: _____ Problem-solving: _____

LIFESTYLE

Habits (coffee, alcohol, smoking): _____

Sleep (quality, number of hours): _____

Meditation/prayer: _____

OTHER NOTES, IMPRESSIONS, FEELINGS

_____

_____

_____

_____

> ***Brain function*** *is intimately tied to our essential*
> *fatty acid intake.*

WEEK 3 / DAY 18   DATE: _____

 EXERCISE FOR THE DAY: *aerobics (20 minutes' vigorous walking)*

WAKE UP: *8-oz glass of water*

MORNING SKIN CARE

DIET

BREAKFAST
- 2 links turkey sausage
- 1 soft-boiled egg
- 1/2 cup slow-cooked oatmeal
- 2-inch wedge cantaloupe
- Green or black tea or water
- 1 Total Skin & Body Vitamin Packet

LUNCH
- 4 ounces chicken salad (diced chicken breast mixed with fresh dill, chopped red onion, chopped celery; dressed with olive oil and lemon juice) served on a bed of romaine lettuce
- 4 hazelnuts
- 1 apple
- Green or black tea or water
- 1 Total Skin & Body Vitamin Packet

AFTERNOON SNACK
- 6 ounces plain whole milk yogurt
- 4 almonds
- 1/4 cup fresh cherries
- Green or black tea or water

DINNER
- 6 ounces broiled fillet of sole, cod, or scrod. (Make 8 ounces and save 2 ounces for tomorrow's bedtime snack.)
- 1 cup steamed spinach
- Romaine lettuce salad with 1/4 cup chickpeas; dressed with olive oil, minced garlic, and lemon juice
- 1/2 cup mixed fresh berries
- Green or black tea or water

BEDTIME SNACK
- 3-ounce can tuna
- 4 macadamia nuts
- 1 pear

EVENING SKIN CARE

RECORD YOUR DAY'S ACTIVITIES, IMPRESSIONS, AND FEELINGS

TAKE A FEW MINUTES TO PRAY, MEDITATE, AND REFLECT

JOURNAL NOTES

THREE THINGS I APPRECIATED IN MY LIFE TODAY:

1. _____
2. _____
3. _____

SKIN

Face and Neck: _____ Fine Lines: _____

Dark Circles: _____ Puffiness: _____

Radiance: _____ Pore Size: _____

Firmness (jawline): _____

BODY

Weight: _____ Tone: _____

Energy: _____ Exercise: _____

MIND

Mood: _____ Stress: _____

Memory: _____ Problem-solving: _____

LIFESTYLE

Habits (coffee, alcohol, smoking): _____

Sleep (quality, number of hours): _____

Meditation/prayer: _____

OTHER NOTES, IMPRESSIONS, FEELINGS

_____

_____

_____

_____

WEEK 3 / DAY 19   DATE: _____

✠ **EXERCISE FOR THE DAY:** *aerobics (20 minutes' vigorous walking)*

💧 **WAKE UP:** *8-oz glass of water*

🧴 **MORNING SKIN CARE**

✗ **DIET**

BREAKFAST
· 3 strips turkey bacon
· $1/2$ cup slow-cooked oatmeal
· 4 hazelnuts
· 2-inch wedge cantaloupe
· Green or black tea or water
· 1 Total Skin & Body Vitamin Packet

LUNCH
· 4 ounces salmon salad (finely cubed salmon fillet or canned salmon dressed with lemon juice, olive oil, and fresh dill) served on a bed of romaine lettuce
· $1/2$ cup lentil soup
· 1 kiwi fruit
· Green or black tea or water
· 1 Total Skin & Body Vitamin Packet

AFTERNOON SNACK
· 2 slices turkey breast
· $1/4$ cup fresh strawberries
· 4 hazelnuts
· Green or black tea or water

DINNER
· 6 ounces baked chicken breast (skin removed)
· $1/2$ cup sautéed zucchini or summer squash topped with 4 chopped almonds
· $1/2$ cup Three Bean Salad*
· 2-inch wedge honeydew melon
· Green or black tea or water

BEDTIME SNACK
· 2 ounces cold fillet of sole, cod, or scrod
· 3 macadamia nuts
· 3 cherry tomatoes

* Recipe available in *The Perricone Prescription: A Physician's 28-Day Program for Total Face and Body Rejuvenation.*

EVENING SKIN CARE

RECORD YOUR DAY'S ACTIVITIES, IMPRESSIONS, AND FEELINGS

TAKE A FEW MINUTES TO PRAY, MEDITATE, AND REFLECT

JOURNAL NOTES

THREE THINGS I APPRECIATED IN MY LIFE TODAY:

1. _____
2. _____
3. _____

SKIN

Face and Neck: _____   Fine Lines: _____

Dark Circles: _____   Puffiness: _____

Radiance: _____   Pore Size: _____

Firmness (jawline): _____

BODY

Weight: _____   Tone: _____

Energy: _____   Exercise: _____

MIND

Mood: _____   Stress: _____

Memory: _____   Problem-solving: _____

LIFESTYLE

Habits (coffee, alcohol, smoking): _____

Sleep (quality, number of hours): _____

Meditation/prayer: _____

OTHER NOTES, IMPRESSIONS, FEELINGS

_____

_____

_____

_____

> *Exercise is vital for your health. Studies have shown that* **exercise benefits the skin** *in much the same way it improves bone and muscle quality.*

WEEK 3 / DAY 20   DATE: _____

EXERCISE FOR THE DAY: *weight training*

 WAKE UP: *8-oz glass of water*

MORNING SKIN CARE

DIET

BREAKFAST
- Omelet made with 2 eggs, 1 ounce crumbled feta cheese, and $1/2$ teaspoon fresh dill
- 2 ounces smoked salmon
- $1/2$ cup blueberries
- Green or black tea or water
- 1 Total Skin & Body Vitamin Packet

LUNCH
- 4 to 6 ounces broiled turkey burger (no bun)
- 1 cup salad made with cherry tomatoes, sliced cucumbers, and chopped red onion; dressed with olive oil and lemon juice
- 1 apple
- Green or black tea or water
- 1 Total Skin & Body Vitamin Packet

AFTERNOON SNACK
- 6 ounces plain whole milk yogurt
- $1/4$ cup sliced fresh strawberries
- Green or black tea or water

DINNER
- 4 to 6 ounces baked or grilled halibut or sea bass
- 1 cup steamed asparagus
- Romaine lettuce salad with $1/4$ cup chickpeas, dressed with olive oil and lemon juice
- 2-inch wedge cantaloupe
- Green or black tea or water

BEDTIME SNACK
- 2 slices roast turkey or chicken breast
- 4 macadamia nuts
- $1/4$ cup fresh cherries

* Recipe available in *The Perricone Prescription: A Physician's 28-Day Program for Total Face and Body Rejuvenation.*

EVENING SKIN CARE

RECORD YOUR DAY'S ACTIVITIES, IMPRESSIONS, AND FEELINGS

TAKE A FEW MINUTES TO PRAY, MEDITATE, AND REFLECT

JOURNAL NOTES

THREE THINGS I APPRECIATED IN MY LIFE TODAY:
1. _____
2. _____
3. _____

SKIN

Face and Neck: _____   Fine Lines: _____

Dark Circles: _____   Puffiness: _____

Radiance: _____   Pore Size: _____

Firmness (jawline): _____

BODY

Weight: _____   Tone: _____

Energy: _____   Exercise: _____

MIND

Mood: _____   Stress: _____

Memory: _____   Problem-solving: _____

LIFESTYLE

Habits (coffee, alcohol, smoking): _____

Sleep (quality, number of hours): _____

Meditation/prayer: _____

OTHER NOTES, IMPRESSIONS, FEELINGS

_____
_____
_____
_____

> *All skin tones are vulnerable to damage from the sun's ultraviolet rays. **Applying sunscreen** at the start of your day should be as automatic as combing your hair.*

WEEK 3 / DAY 21　　　　DATE: _____

 EXERCISE FOR THE DAY: *relaxation*

WAKE UP: *8-oz glass of water*

MORNING SKIN CARE

DIET

BREAKFAST
- 3 ounces broiled salmon
- 1/2 cup slow-cooked oatmeal
- 2-inch wedge cantaloupe
- Green or black tea or water
- 1 Total Skin & Body Vitamin Packet

LUNCH
- 6-ounce can of tuna or sardines
- Greek salad with romaine lettuce, 3 black olives, 1 ounce feta cheese, 1/2 sliced cucumber, 4 cherry tomatoes; dress with olive oil, lemon juice, dash of oregano; toss
- 1/2 cup mixed fresh berries
- Green or black tea or water
- 1 Total Skin & Body Vitamin Packet

AFTERNOON SNACK
- 1/2 cup plain cottage cheese
- 4 hazelnuts
- 1 apple
- Green or black tea or water

DINNER
- Chicken Stir Fry (6 ounces chicken breast chopped into 1-inch strips; 1/4 cup each sliced mushrooms, chopped onions, water chestnuts, chopped almonds, bamboo shoots, bok choy or celery, and mung bean sprouts; toss together and stir fry in olive oil)
- Romaine lettuce salad dressed with olive oil and lemon juice
- 2-inch wedge cantaloupe
- Green or black tea or water

BEDTIME SNACK
- 2 slices turkey breast
- 3 olives
- 1 pear

EVENING SKIN CARE

RECORD YOUR DAY'S ACTIVITIES, IMPRESSIONS, AND FEELINGS

TAKE A FEW MINUTES TO PRAY, MEDITATE, AND REFLECT

JOURNAL NOTES

THREE THINGS I APPRECIATED IN MY LIFE TODAY:

1. _____
2. _____
3. _____

SKIN

Face and Neck: _____   Fine Lines: _____

Dark Circles: _____   Puffiness: _____

Radiance: _____   Pore Size: _____

Firmness (jawline): _____

BODY

Weight: _____   Tone: _____

Energy: _____   Exercise: _____

MIND

Mood: _____   Stress: _____

Memory: _____   Problem-solving: _____

LIFESTYLE

Habits (coffee, alcohol, smoking): _____

Sleep (quality, number of hours): _____

Meditation/prayer: _____

OTHER NOTES, IMPRESSIONS, FEELINGS

_____

_____

_____

_____

*Food is much more than just a life-giving and life-sustaining substance—it is our **single most powerful** anti-aging tool.*

WEEK 4 / DAY 22   DATE: _____

EXERCISE FOR THE DAY: *aerobics (20 minutes' vigorous walking)*

WAKE UP: *8-oz glass of water*

MORNING SKIN CARE

DIET

BREAKFAST
- 2 links turkey sausage
- 1 soft-boiled egg
- 1/2 grapefruit
- Green or black tea or water
- 1 Total Skin & Body Vitamin Packet

LUNCH
- 6-ounce canned crabmeat mixed with 1 teaspoon mayonnaise and 1 chopped celery stalk
- 1/2 cup lentil soup
- 1 apple
- Green or black tea or water
- 1 Total Skin & Body Vitamin Packet

AFTERNOON SNACK
- 2 ounces smoked salmon
- 2-inch wedge cantaloupe
- Green or black tea or water

DINNER
- 6 ounces scallops sautéed with minced garlic in olive oil. (Cook 8 ounces and save 2 ounces for tomorrow's lunch.)
- 1/2 cup steamed broccoli
- 1/4 cup fresh cherries
- Green or black tea or water

BEDTIME SNACK
- 6 ounces plain whole milk yogurt
- 4 hazelnuts
- 1/4 cup blueberries

JOURNAL NOTES

THREE THINGS I APPRECIATED IN MY LIFE TODAY:
1. _____
2. _____
3. _____

SKIN

Face and Neck: _____   Fine Lines: _____

Dark Circles: _____   Puffiness: _____

Radiance: _____   Pore Size: _____

Firmness (jawline): _____

BODY

Weight: _____   Tone: _____

Energy: _____   Exercise: _____

MIND

Mood: _____   Stress: _____

Memory: _____   Problem-solving: _____

LIFESTYLE

Habits (coffee, alcohol, smoking): _____

Sleep (quality, number of hours): _____

Meditation/prayer: _____

OTHER NOTES, IMPRESSIONS, FEELINGS

_____

_____

_____

_____

> *The **fountain of youth** did not spew forth diet soda or orange juice—it's always been good old H$_2$0.*

WEEK 4 / DAY 23   DATE: _____

EXERCISE FOR THE DAY: *weight training*

WAKE UP: *8-oz glass of water*

MORNING SKIN CARE

DIET

BREAKFAST
- Vegetable omelet made with 2 eggs and $1/4$ cup each chopped onions, sliced mushrooms, and chopped green pepper
- $1/2$ cup slow-cooked oatmeal
- 3 hazelnuts
- $1/2$ grapefruit
- Green or black tea or water
- 1 Total Skin & Body Vitamin Packet

LUNCH
- Scallop salad made with 2 ounces scallops (from previous night's dinner), chopped red onion, 3 chopped black olives and fresh dill, dressed with olive oil and lemon juice
- 2-inch wedge honeydew melon
- Green or black tea or water
- 1 Total Skin & Body Vitamin Packet

AFTERNOON SNACK
- 6 ounces plain whole milk yogurt
- $1/4$ cup fresh blueberries, blackberries, or raspberries
- 3 macadamia nuts
- Green or black tea or water

DINNER
- 6 ounces grilled salmon
- $1/2$ cup lentil soup
- Romaine lettuce salad dressed with olive oil and lemon juice
- $1/2$ cup fresh cherries
- Green or black tea or water

BEDTIME SNACK
- $1/2$ cup plain cottage cheese
- 3 strawberries
- 4 hazelnuts

EVENING SKIN CARE

RECORD YOUR DAY'S ACTIVITIES, IMPRESSIONS, AND FEELINGS

TAKE A FEW MINUTES TO PRAY, MEDITATE, AND REFLECT

JOURNAL NOTES

THREE THINGS I APPRECIATED IN MY LIFE TODAY:
1. _____
2. _____
3. _____

SKIN

Face and Neck: _____   Fine Lines: _____

Dark Circles: _____   Puffiness: _____

Radiance: _____   Pore Size: _____

Firmness (jawline): _____

BODY

Weight: _____   Tone: _____

Energy: _____   Exercise: _____

MIND

Mood: _____   Stress: _____

Memory: _____   Problem-solving: _____

LIFESTYLE

Habits (coffee, alcohol, smoking): _____

Sleep (quality, number of hours): _____

Meditation/prayer: _____

OTHER NOTES, IMPRESSIONS, FEELINGS

_____

_____

_____

_____

WEEK 4 / DAY 24   DATE: _____

✚ **EXERCISE FOR THE DAY:** *aerobics (20 minutes' vigorous walking)*

💧 **WAKE UP:** *8-oz glass of water*

🧴 **MORNING SKIN CARE**

✗ **DIET**

BREAKFAST
· 2 links turkey sausage
· 1 poached egg
· 3 almonds
· 2-inch wedge cantaloupe
· Green or black tea or water
· 1 Total Skin & Body Vitamin Packet

LUNCH
· 4 to 6 ounces grilled chicken breast
· Romaine lettuce salad with sliced tomatoes and $1/4$ cup chickpeas;
  dressed with olive oil and lemon juice
· $1/2$ cup fresh cherries
· Green or black tea or water
· 1 Total Skin & Body Vitamin Packet

AFTERNOON SNACK
· 6 ounces plain whole milk yogurt
· 4 hazelnuts
· 1 kiwi fruit
· Green or black tea or water

DINNER
· 6 ounces broiled trout
· Mixed three-leaf salad (arugula, radicchio, and endive) dressed with
  olive oil and lemon juice
· $1/2$ cup green beans garnished with chopped almonds
· Green or black tea or water

BEDTIME SNACK
· 2 slices chicken or turkey breast
· 4 macadamia nuts
· 1 small pear

EVENING SKIN CARE

RECORD YOUR DAY'S ACTIVITIES, IMPRESSIONS, AND FEELINGS

TAKE A FEW MINUTES TO PRAY, MEDITATE, AND REFLECT

JOURNAL NOTES

THREE THINGS I APPRECIATED IN MY LIFE TODAY:

1. _____

2. _____

3. _____

SKIN

Face and Neck: _____   Fine Lines: _____

Dark Circles: _____   Puffiness: _____

Radiance: _____   Pore Size: _____

Firmness (jawline): _____

BODY

Weight: _____   Tone: _____

Energy: _____   Exercise: _____

MIND

Mood: _____   Stress: _____

Memory: _____   Problem-solving: _____

LIFESTYLE

Habits (coffee, alcohol, smoking): _____

Sleep (quality, number of hours): _____

Meditation/prayer: _____

OTHER NOTES, IMPRESSIONS, FEELINGS

_____

_____

_____

_____

WEEK 4 / DAY 25   DATE: _____

EXERCISE FOR THE DAY: *weight training*

WAKE UP: *8-oz glass of water*

MORNING SKIN CARE

DIET

BREAKFAST
- 4 ounces smoked salmon
- 1 slice tomato
- $1/2$ grapefruit
- Green or black tea or water
- 1 Total Skin & Body Vitamin Packet

LUNCH
- Crabmeat salad (1 6-ounce can of crabmeat mixed with 1 chopped scallion, 1 chopped celery rib, $1/4$ cup plain yogurt and juice of $1/2$ lemon) served inside $1/2$ avocado
- $1/2$ cup lentil soup
- Green or black tea or water
- 1 Total Skin & Body Vitamin Packet

AFTERNOON SNACK
- 1 hard-boiled egg
- 4 cherry tomatoes
- 4 macadamia nuts
- Green or black tea or water

DINNER
- 6 ounces baked turkey breast.
- 1 small eggplant, sliced and grilled, topped with sliced tomato and 1 tablespoon grated Parmesan cheese
- 1 apple
- Green or black tea or water

BEDTIME SNACK
- 6 ounces plain whole milk yogurt
- 4 hazelnuts
- $1/4$ cup blueberries

EVENING SKIN CARE

RECORD YOUR DAY'S ACTIVITIES, IMPRESSIONS, AND FEELINGS

TAKE A FEW MINUTES TO PRAY, MEDITATE, AND REFLECT

JOURNAL NOTES

THREE THINGS I APPRECIATED IN MY LIFE TODAY:

1. _____

2. _____

3. _____

SKIN

Face and Neck: _____   Fine Lines: _____

Dark Circles: _____   Puffiness: _____

Radiance: _____   Pore Size: _____

Firmness (jawline): _____

BODY

Weight: _____   Tone: _____

Energy: _____   Exercise: _____

MIND

Mood: _____   Stress: _____

Memory: _____   Problem-solving: _____

LIFESTYLE

Habits (coffee, alcohol, smoking): _____

Sleep (quality, number of hours): _____

Meditation/prayer: _____

OTHER NOTES, IMPRESSIONS, FEELINGS

_____

_____

_____

_____

WEEK 4 / DAY 26   DATE: _____

EXERCISE FOR THE DAY: *aerobics (20 minutes' vigorous walking)*

WAKE UP: *8-oz glass of water*

MORNING SKIN CARE

DIET

BREAKFAST
· 2 slices turkey bacon
· 2 soft-boiled eggs
· 2-inch wedge cantaloupe
· Green or black tea or water
· 1 Total Skin & Body Vitamin Packet

LUNCH
· 3 to 5 ounces chicken salad (mix 2 ounces chicken saved from last night's dinner with 1 teaspoon each chopped red onion and celery, 4 chopped hazelnuts, and 1 tablespoon olive oil and lemon juice) served on a bed of romaine lettuce
· 1 pear
· Green or black tea or water
· 1 Total Skin & Body Vitamin Packet

AFTERNOON SNACK
· 6 ounces plain whole milk yogurt
· $1/4$ cup fresh cherries
· 4 hazelnuts
· Green or black tea or water

DINNER
· 6 ounces grilled salmon
· Salad of romaine lettuce, avocado, and tomato, dressed with olive oil and lemon juice
· 1 cup steamed asparagus
· Green or black tea or water

BEDTIME SNACK
· 2 ounces tuna
· 4 green or black olives
· $1/4$ cup blueberries

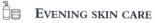 **EVENING SKIN CARE**

RECORD YOUR DAY'S ACTIVITIES, IMPRESSIONS, AND FEELINGS

TAKE A FEW MINUTES TO PRAY, MEDITATE, AND REFLECT

JOURNAL NOTES

THREE THINGS I APPRECIATED IN MY LIFE TODAY:

1. _____

2. _____

3. _____

SKIN

Face and Neck: _____   Fine Lines: _____

Dark Circles: _____   Puffiness: _____

Radiance: _____   Pore Size: _____

Firmness (jawline): _____

BODY

Weight: _____   Tone: _____

Energy: _____   Exercise: _____

MIND

Mood: _____   Stress: _____

Memory: _____   Problem-solving: _____

LIFESTYLE

Habits (coffee, alcohol, smoking): _____

Sleep (quality, number of hours): _____

Meditation/prayer: _____

OTHER NOTES, IMPRESSIONS, FEELINGS

_____

_____

_____

_____

> *Researchers in Boston found patients with manic-depressive disorder who had not responded to conventional treatment **improved dramatically** when given a daily four-ounce serving of salmon.*

WEEK 4 / DAY 27   DATE: _____

EXERCISE FOR THE DAY: *aerobics*

WAKE UP: *8-oz glass of water*

MORNING SKIN CARE

DIET

BREAKFAST
- 2 to 4 ounces smoked salmon
- 6 ounces plain whole milk yogurt
- 4 chopped walnuts
- 1/2 grapefruit
- Green or black tea or water
- 1 Total Skin & Body Vitamin Packet

LUNCH
- 6 ounces grilled turkey burger topped with romaine lettuce, sliced tomato, alfalfa sprouts, and red onion (no bun)
- 1/2 cup lentil soup
- 2-inch wedge honeydew melon
- Green or black tea or water
- 1 Total Skin & Body Vitamin Packet

AFTERNOON SNACK
- 2 ounces sliced chicken breast
- 2-inch wedge cantaloupe
- 4 macadamia nuts
- Green or black tea or water

DINNER
- 6 ounces grilled bluefin or albacore tuna steak
- 1 cup steamed spinach
- Romaine lettuce salad tossed with olive oil and lemon juice
- 1/4 cup mixed fresh berries
- Green or black tea or water

BEDTIME SNACK
- 2 slices turkey breast
- 4 green olives
- 4 cherry tomatoes

EVENING SKIN CARE

RECORD YOUR DAY'S ACTIVITIES, IMPRESSIONS, AND FEELINGS

TAKE A FEW MINUTES TO PRAY, MEDITATE, AND REFLECT

JOURNAL NOTES

THREE THINGS I APPRECIATED IN MY LIFE TODAY:
1. _____
2. _____
3. _____

SKIN

Face and Neck: _____   Fine Lines: _____

Dark Circles: _____   Puffiness: _____

Radiance: _____   Pore Size: _____

Firmness (jawline): _____

BODY

Weight: _____   Tone: _____

Energy: _____   Exercise: _____

MIND

Mood: _____   Stress: _____

Memory: _____   Problem-solving: _____

LIFESTYLE

Habits (coffee, alcohol, smoking): _____

Sleep (quality, number of hours): _____

Meditation/prayer: _____

OTHER NOTES, IMPRESSIONS, FEELINGS

_____
_____
_____
_____

> *Once you accept that your **everyday lifestyle choices**
> affect the way you age, you are on your way toward
> restoring youthful looks and vigor.*

WEEK 4 / DAY 28　　　DATE: _____

 EXERCISE FOR THE DAY: *relaxation*

WAKE UP: *8-oz glass of water*

MORNING SKIN CARE

DIET

BREAKFAST
- 2 ounces smoked salmon
- $1/2$ cup slow-cooked oatmeal
- 2-inch wedge cantaloupe
- Green or black tea or water
- 1 Total Skin & Body Vitamin Packet

LUNCH
- 3 to 4 ounces tuna tossed with $1/2$ cup white beans, 4 cherry tomatoes, and sliced red onion; dress with olive oil and lemon juice and serve on a bed of romaine lettuce
- 1 apple
- Green or black tea or water
- 1 Total Skin & Body Vitamin Packet

AFTERNOON SNACK
- 6 ounces plain whole milk yogurt
- 4 hazelnuts
- $1/2$ grapefruit
- Green or black tea or water

DINNER
- 4 large shrimp, brushed with olive oil and baked
- Salad of romaine lettuce, $1/4$ cup chickpeas, chopped celery, sliced tomato, and sliced avocado; dress with oil and lemon juice
- $1/4$ cup mixed fresh berries
- Green or black tea or water

BEDTIME SNACK
- $1/2$ cup cottage cheese
- 4 hazelnuts
- 1 pear

EVENING SKIN CARE

RECORD YOUR DAY'S ACTIVITIES, IMPRESSIONS, AND FEELINGS

TAKE A FEW MINUTES TO PRAY, MEDITATE, AND REFLECT

JOURNAL NOTES

THREE THINGS I APPRECIATED IN MY LIFE TODAY:
1. _____
2. _____
3. _____

SKIN

Face and Neck: _____   Fine Lines: _____

Dark Circles: _____   Puffiness: _____

Radiance: _____   Pore Size: _____

Firmness (jawline): _____

BODY

Weight: _____   Tone: _____

Energy: _____   Exercise: _____

MIND

Mood: _____   Stress: _____

Memory: _____   Problem-solving: _____

LIFESTYLE

Habits (coffee, alcohol, smoking): _____

Sleep (quality, number of hours): _____

Meditation/prayer: _____

OTHER NOTES, IMPRESSIONS, FEELINGS

_____

_____

_____

_____

WEEK 5 / DAY 29   DATE: _____

EXERCISE FOR THE DAY: *aerobics*

WAKE UP: *8-oz glass of water*

MORNING SKIN CARE

DIET

BREAKFAST
- 3 to 4 ounces smoked Nova Scotia salmon
- 1/2 cup slow-cooked oatmeal with 2 tablespoons blueberries
- 1 teaspoon slivered almonds
- Green or black tea or water
- 1 Total Skin & Body Vitamin Packet

LUNCH
- 4- to 6-ounce broiled turkey burger (no bun)
- Lettuce and tomato
- 1/2 cup Three-Bean Salad*
- Green or black tea or water
- 1 Total Skin & Body Vitamin Packet

AFTERNOON SNACK
- 2 ounces sliced turkey or chicken breast
- 4 hazelnuts
- 4 celery sticks
- Green or black tea or water

DINNER
- 4 to 6 ounces broiled salmon
- 1 cup lentil soup
- Tossed green salad dressed with olive oil and lemon juice
- 1/2 cup steamed spinach
- Green or black tea or water

BEDTIME SNACK
- 1 hard-boiled egg
- 3 celery sticks
- 3 red bell pepper strips
- 3 green olives

* Recipe available in *The Perricone Prescription: A Physician's 28-Day Program for Total Face and Body Rejuvenation.*

- **EVENING SKIN CARE**
- **RECORD YOUR DAY'S ACTIVITIES, IMPRESSIONS, AND FEELINGS**
- **TAKE A FEW MINUTES TO PRAY, MEDITATE, AND REFLECT**

JOURNAL NOTES

THREE THINGS I APPRECIATED IN MY LIFE TODAY:
1. _____
2. _____
3. _____

SKIN

Face and Neck: _____   Fine Lines: _____

Dark Circles: _____   Puffiness: _____

Radiance: _____   Pore Size: _____

Firmness (jawline): _____

BODY

Weight: _____   Tone: _____

Energy: _____   Exercise: _____

MIND

Mood: _____   Stress: _____

Memory: _____   Problem-solving: _____

LIFESTYLE

Habits (coffee, alcohol, smoking): _____

Sleep (quality, number of hours): _____

Meditation/prayer: _____

OTHER NOTES, IMPRESSIONS, FEELINGS

_____

_____

_____

_____

WEEK 5 / DAY 30   DATE: _____

EXERCISE FOR THE DAY: *weight training*

WAKE UP: *8-oz glass of water*

MORNING SKIN CARE

DIET

BREAKFAST
· Omelet made with 3 egg whites and one yolk
· Sliced tomato
· 1/2 cup blueberries
· Green or black tea or water
· 1 Total Skin & Body Vitamin Packet

LUNCH
· 3 to 6 ounces smoked or grilled salmon
· Green salad with tomatoes, cucumbers, onions and 2 tablespoons chickpeas dressed with olive oil, lemon juice, and garlic
· Green or black tea or water
· 1 Total Skin & Body Vitamin Packet

AFTERNOON SNACK
· 1/2 cup low-fat cottage cheese
· 4 small black olives
· 4 endive spears
· Green or black tea or water

DINNER
· 4 to 6 ounces baked or grilled halibut
· 1 cup Chicken-Vegetable Soup*
· Salad of romaine lettuce, chopped avocado, tomato, green onion, and celery dressed with olive oil and lemon juice
· Green or black tea or water

BEDTIME SNACK
· 2 ounces sliced roast turkey breast
· 6 whole almonds
· 3 red bell pepper strips
· 2-inch wedge of honeydew melon

* Recipe available in *The Perricone Prescription: A Physician's 28-Day Program for Total Face and Body Rejuvenation.*

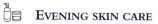

Evening skin care

Record your day's activities, impressions, and feelings

Take a few minutes to pray, meditate, and reflect

Journal Notes

THREE THINGS I APPRECIATED IN MY LIFE TODAY:

1. _____
2. _____
3. _____

SKIN

Face and Neck: _____   Fine Lines: _____

Dark Circles: _____   Puffiness: _____

Radiance: _____   Pore Size: _____

Firmness (jawline): _____

BODY

Weight: _____   Tone: _____

Energy: _____   Exercise: _____

MIND

Mood: _____   Stress: _____

Memory: _____   Problem-solving: _____

LIFESTYLE

Habits (coffee, alcohol, smoking): _____

Sleep (quality, number of hours): _____

Meditation/prayer: _____

OTHER NOTES, IMPRESSIONS, FEELINGS

_____

_____

_____

_____

WEEK 5 / DAY 31   DATE: _____

 EXERCISE FOR THE DAY: *aerobics*

 WAKE UP: *8-oz glass of water*

MORNING SKIN CARE

DIET

BREAKFAST
- 2 slices turkey bacon
- 6 ounces plain whole milk yogurt
- ¹/₂ cup strawberries
- Green or black tea or water
- 1 Total Skin & Body Vitamin Packet

LUNCH
- 3- to 4-ounce can water-packed tuna
- 1 cup sliced tomatoes and cucumbers
- ¹/₂ cup bean salad
- Green or black tea or water
- 1 Total Skin & Body Vitamin Packet

AFTERNOON SNACK
- 2 ounces sliced turkey breast
- 4 hazelnuts
- 1 small pear
- Green or black tea or water

DINNER
- 4 to 6 ounces broiled fillet of salmon. (Make 8 ounces and save 2 ounces for tomorrow's bedtime snack.)
- ¹/₄ cup green beans
- Spinach salad with mushrooms, slice of red onion, and ¹/₄ cup chickpeas, dressed with olive oil and lemon juice
- Green or black tea or water

BEDTIME SNACK
- 2 ounces Grilled Chicken Breast*
- ¹/₄ cup raw cauliflower
- 4 black olives

* Recipe available in *The Perricone Prescription: A Physician's 28-Day Program for Total Face and Body Rejuvenation.*

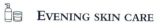

EVENING SKIN CARE

RECORD YOUR DAY'S ACTIVITIES, IMPRESSIONS, AND FEELINGS

TAKE A FEW MINUTES TO PRAY, MEDITATE, AND REFLECT

JOURNAL NOTES

THREE THINGS I APPRECIATED IN MY LIFE TODAY:

1. _____

2. _____

3. _____

SKIN

Face and Neck: _____   Fine Lines: _____

Dark Circles: _____   Puffiness: _____

Radiance: _____   Pore Size: _____

Firmness (jawline): _____

BODY

Weight: _____   Tone: _____

Energy: _____   Exercise: _____

MIND

Mood: _____   Stress: _____

Memory: _____   Problem-solving: _____

LIFESTYLE

Habits (coffee, alcohol, smoking): _____

Sleep (quality, number of hours): _____

Meditation/prayer: _____

OTHER NOTES, IMPRESSIONS, FEELINGS

_____

_____

_____

_____

> *Exercise in moderation has a **powerful, positive and anti-inflammatory** effect on our cells.*

WEEK 5 / DAY 32   DATE: _____

 EXERCISE FOR THE DAY: *weight training*

WAKE UP: *8-oz glass of water*

MORNING SKIN CARE

DIET

BREAKFAST
· 1 slice of Canadian bacon or 2 slices turkey bacon
· 2 poached egg whites and one yolk
· ¹/₂ cup slow-cooked oatmeal
· ¹/₂ cup blueberries
· Green or black tea or water
· 1 Total Skin & Body Vitamin Packet

LUNCH
· 4 ounces grilled chicken salad (with fresh dill, chopped red onion, garlic, and olive oil)
· ¹/₂ cup steamed broccoli
· ¹/₂ cup strawberries
· Green or black tea or water
· 1 Total Skin & Body Vitamin Packet

AFTERNOON SNACK
· 2 slices roast turkey breast
· 4 cherry tomatoes
· 4 almonds
· Green or black tea or water

DINNER
· 6 ounces broiled fillet of sole, cod, or scrod.
· 8 Oven-Roasted Brussels Sprouts with Apples*
· Romaine lettuce salad with 2 ounces chickpeas, dressed with olive oil, garlic, and lemon juice
· Green or black tea or water

BEDTIME SNACK
· 2 ounces salmon
· 2 tablespoons Cuban Black Bean Salad*

* Recipe available in *The Perricone Prescription: A Physician's 28-Day Program for Total Face and Body Rejuvenation.*

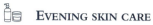 **E**VENING SKIN CARE

RECORD YOUR DAY'S ACTIVITIES, IMPRESSIONS, AND FEELINGS

TAKE A FEW MINUTES TO PRAY, MEDITATE, AND REFLECT

JOURNAL NOTES

THREE THINGS I APPRECIATED IN MY LIFE TODAY:

1. _____

2. _____

3. _____

SKIN

Face and Neck: _____   Fine Lines: _____

Dark Circles: _____   Puffiness: _____

Radiance: _____   Pore Size: _____

Firmness (jawline): _____

BODY

Weight: _____   Tone: _____

Energy: _____   Exercise: _____

MIND

Mood: _____   Stress: _____

Memory: _____   Problem-solving: _____

LIFESTYLE

Habits (coffee, alcohol, smoking): _____

Sleep (quality, number of hours): _____

Meditation/prayer: _____

OTHER NOTES, IMPRESSIONS, FEELINGS

_____

_____

_____

_____

WEEK 5 / DAY 33   DATE: _____

EXERCISE FOR THE DAY: *aerobics (20 minutes' vigorous walking)*

WAKE UP: *8-oz glass of water*

MORNING SKIN CARE

DIET

BREAKFAST
- 4 ounces smoked salmon
- 1/2 cup slow-cooked oatmeal seasoned with cinnamon
- 2 teaspoons chopped almonds
- 2-inch wedge of cantaloupe
- Green or black tea or water
- 1 Total Skin & Body Vitamin Packet

LUNCH
- 4 ounces salmon salad (finely cubed salmon fillet or canned salmon dressed with lemon juice, olive oil, and dill) served on a bed of romaine lettuce
- 1/2 cup lentil soup
- Green or black tea or water
- 1 Total Skin & Body Vitamin Packet

AFTERNOON SNACK
- 2 slices turkey breast
- 1/2 cup strawberries
- 4 hazelnuts
- Green or black tea or water

DINNER
- 1 roast chicken breast (skin removed)
- 1/2 cup grilled zucchini
- 1/2 cup Three Bean Salad*
- Green or black tea or water

BEDTIME SNACK
- 2 ounces drained canned shrimp or tuna
- 3 macadamia nuts
- 3 cherry tomatoes

* Recipe available in *The Perricone Prescription: A Physician's 28-Day Program for Total Face and Body Rejuvenation.*

JOURNAL NOTES

THREE THINGS I APPRECIATED IN MY LIFE TODAY:

1. _____
2. _____
3. _____

SKIN

Face and Neck: _____   Fine Lines: _____

Dark Circles: _____   Puffiness: _____

Radiance: _____   Pore Size: _____

Firmness (jawline): _____

BODY

Weight: _____   Tone: _____

Energy: _____   Exercise: _____

MIND

Mood: _____   Stress: _____

Memory: _____   Problem-solving: _____

LIFESTYLE

Habits (coffee, alcohol, smoking): _____

Sleep (quality, number of hours): _____

Meditation/prayer: _____

OTHER NOTES, IMPRESSIONS, FEELINGS

_____
_____
_____
_____

> *Not all fats are bad—and **the right fats** can help you lose weight.*

WEEK 5 / DAY 34   DATE: _____

 EXERCISE FOR THE DAY: *weight training*

WAKE UP: *8-oz glass of water*

MORNING SKIN CARE

DIET

BREAKFAST
- Omelet of 3 egg whites and 1 yolk with a few sliced mushrooms and 1/2 cup chopped spinach
- 1 slice Canadian or turkey bacon
- 2-inch wedge of honeydew melon
- Green or black tea or water
- 1 Total Skin & Body Vitamin Packet

LUNCH
- 4 to 6 ounces broiled salmon
- Caesar salad without croutons
- 1/2 apple
- Green or black tea or water
- 1 Total Skin & Body Vitamin Packet

AFTERNOON SNACK
- 1 hard-boiled egg
- 1/2 cup sliced strawberries
- 3 almonds
- Green or black tea or water

DINNER
- 4 to 6 ounces grilled halibut
- Tossed Greek salad made with romaine lettuce, 3 black olives, 1 ounce feta cheese, 1/2 cucumber, 4 cherry tomatoes; dressed with olive oil, lemon juice, and a dash of oregano, mixed to taste
- Steamed or Grilled Asparagus*
- 2-inch wedge of cataloupe
- Green or black tea or water

BEDTIME SNACK
- 2 slices roast turkey or chicken breast
- 4 macadamia nuts
- Small peach or nectarine

* Recipe available in *The Perricone Prescription: A Physician's 28-Day Program for Total Face and Body Rejuvenation.*

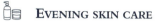 **Evening skin care**

Record your day's activities, impressions, and feelings

Take a few minutes to pray, meditate, and reflect

Journal Notes

THREE THINGS I APPRECIATED IN MY LIFE TODAY:

1. _____
2. _____
3. _____

SKIN

Face and Neck: _____   Fine Lines: _____

Dark Circles: _____   Puffiness: _____

Radiance: _____   Pore Size: _____

Firmness (jawline): _____

BODY

Weight: _____   Tone: _____

Energy: _____   Exercise: _____

MIND

Mood: _____   Stress: _____

Memory: _____   Problem-solving: _____

LIFESTYLE

Habits (coffee, alcohol, smoking): _____

Sleep (quality, number of hours): _____

Meditation/prayer: _____

OTHER NOTES, IMPRESSIONS, FEELINGS

_____

_____

_____

_____

> *A diet rich in **extra virgin olive oil** increases the skin's ability to maintain moisture, lowers blood pressure, prevents osteoporosis, reduces the risk of certain cancers... and much more.*

WEEK 5 / DAY 35   DATE: _____

EXERCISE FOR THE DAY: *relaxation (you've earned it!)*

WAKE UP: *8-oz glass of water*

MORNING SKIN CARE

DIET

BREAKFAST
· 3 to 6 ounces broiled salmon
· $1/2$ cup slow-cooked oatmeal
· 2-inch wedge of cantaloupe
· Green or black tea or water
· 1 Total Skin & Body Vitamin Packet

LUNCH
· Crabmeat salad made with a 6-ounce can of crabmeat, 1 chopped scallion, 1 chopped celery rib; dress with $1/4$ cup yogurt, juice of $1/2$ lemon; serve inside $1/2$ avocado
· 1 cup strawberries
· Green or black tea or water
· 1 Total Skin & Body Vitamin Packet

AFTERNOON SNACK
· $1/2$ cup cottage cheese
· 4 almonds
· 1 apple
· Green or black tea or water

DINNER
· Grilled chicken breast*
· $3/4$ cup roasted or sautéed mushrooms and Sautéed Zucchini or Summer Squash*
· Romaine lettuce salad, sliced tomatoes, fresh basil with 1 ounce grated Parmesan cheese, dressed with olive oil and lemon juice, mixed to taste
· Green or black tea or water

BEDTIME SNACK
· 2 slices of turkey breast
· 3 olives
· 1 pear

* Recipe available in *The Perricone Prescription: A Physician's 28-Day Program for Total Face and Body Rejuvenation.*

EVENING SKIN CARE

RECORD YOUR DAY'S ACTIVITIES, IMPRESSIONS, AND FEELINGS

TAKE A FEW MINUTES TO PRAY, MEDITATE, AND REFLECT

JOURNAL NOTES

THREE THINGS I APPRECIATED IN MY LIFE TODAY:
1. _____
2. _____
3. _____

SKIN

Face and Neck: _____   Fine Lines: _____

Dark Circles: _____   Puffiness: _____

Radiance: _____   Pore Size: _____

Firmness (jawline): _____

BODY

Weight: _____   Tone: _____

Energy: _____   Exercise: _____

MIND

Mood: _____   Stress: _____

Memory: _____   Problem-solving: _____

LIFESTYLE

Habits (coffee, alcohol, smoking): _____

Sleep (quality, number of hours): _____

Meditation/prayer: _____

OTHER NOTES, IMPRESSIONS, FEELINGS

_____
_____
_____
_____

> *Alpha lipoic acid is a **natural substance** found in our bodies—and it is one of the most powerful anti-aging, antioxidant, anti-inflammatories available.*

WEEK 6 / DAY 36   DATE: _____

EXERCISE FOR THE DAY: *aerobics (20 minutes' vigorous walking)*

WAKE UP: *8-oz glass of water*

MORNING SKIN CARE

DIET

BREAKFAST
· 2 slices Canadian bacon, ham, or turkey bacon
· 1/2 cup plain cottage cheese
· 1/2 cup blueberries
· Green or black tea or water
· 1 Total Skin & Body Vitamin Packet

LUNCH
· 3- to 4-ounce can water-packed tuna
· 1/2 cup lentil soup
· Romaine lettuce salad topped with chopped tomato and red onion; dress with olive oil and lemon
· Green or black tea or water
· 1 Total Skin & Body Vitamin Packet

AFTERNOON SNACK
· 2 ounces smoked salmon
· 3 hazelnuts
· 2-inch wedge cantaloupe
· Green or black tea or water

DINNER
· 6 ounces Scallops with Garlic and Parsley* (cook 8 ounces and save 2 ounces for tomorrow's lunch)
· Mediterranean Chopped Salad* with 1/2 cup chickpeas
· 1/2 cup cooked green beans
· Green or black tea or water

BEDTIME SNACK
· 2 slices turkey breast
· 4 green olives
· 1 apple

* Recipe available in *The Perricone Prescription: A Physician's 28-Day Program for Total Face and Body Rejuvenation.*

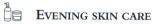

EVENING SKIN CARE

RECORD YOUR DAY'S ACTIVITIES, IMPRESSIONS, AND FEELINGS

TAKE A FEW MINUTES TO PRAY, MEDITATE, AND REFLECT

JOURNAL NOTES

THREE THINGS I APPRECIATED IN MY LIFE TODAY:
1. _____
2. _____
3. _____

SKIN

Face and Neck: _____   Fine Lines: _____

Dark Circles: _____   Puffiness: _____

Radiance: _____   Pore Size: _____

Firmness (jawline): _____

BODY

Weight: _____   Tone: _____

Energy: _____   Exercise: _____

MIND

Mood: _____   Stress: _____

Memory: _____   Problem-solving: _____

LIFESTYLE

Habits (coffee, alcohol, smoking): _____

Sleep (quality, number of hours): _____

Meditation/prayer: _____

OTHER NOTES, IMPRESSIONS, FEELINGS

_____

_____

_____

_____

> *Even the busiest person can find time during the day*
> *for a **twenty-minute walk**.*

Week 6 / Day 37   Date: _____

 Exercise for the day: *weight training*

Wake up: *8-oz glass of water*

Morning skin care

Diet

BREAKFAST
· Egg white omelet made with 3 to 4 egg whites and one yolk (add a few sliced mushrooms, if desired)
· 1/2 cup slow-cooked oatmeal
· 3 hazelnuts
· Green or black tea or water
· 1 Total Skin & Body Vitamin Packet

LUNCH
· Scallop salad (2 ounces scallops from previous night's dinner); dressed with olive oil, lemon juice, chopped red onion, and dill
· 1/2 cup Three Bean Salad*
· Green or black tea or water
· 1 Total Skin & Body Vitamin Packet

AFTERNOON SNACK
· 2 ounces smoked salmon
· 4 black olives
· 3 endive spears
· Green or black tea or water

DINNER
· 6 ounces grilled salmon
· 1/2 cup Cuban Black Bean Soup*
· Romaine salad dressed with olive oil and lemon juice
· 1/2 cup berries
· Green or black tea or water

BEDTIME SNACK
· 6 ounces plain whole milk yogurt or cottage cheese
· 1/2 cup strawberries
· 4 macadamia nuts

* Recipe available in *The Perricone Prescription: A Physician's 28-Day Program for Total Face and Body Rejuvenation.*

EVENING SKIN CARE

RECORD YOUR DAY'S ACTIVITIES, IMPRESSIONS, AND FEELINGS

TAKE A FEW MINUTES TO PRAY, MEDITATE, AND REFLECT

JOURNAL NOTES

THREE THINGS I APPRECIATED IN MY LIFE TODAY:

1. _____
2. _____
3. _____

SKIN

Face and Neck: _____   Fine Lines: _____

Dark Circles: _____   Puffiness: _____

Radiance: _____   Pore Size: _____

Firmness (jawline): _____

BODY

Weight: _____   Tone: _____

Energy: _____   Exercise: _____

MIND

Mood: _____   Stress: _____

Memory: _____   Problem-solving: _____

LIFESTYLE

Habits (coffee, alcohol, smoking): _____

Sleep (quality, number of hours): _____

Meditation/prayer: _____

OTHER NOTES, IMPRESSIONS, FEELINGS

_____

_____

_____

_____

WEEK 6 / DAY 38   DATE: _____

 EXERCISE FOR THE DAY: *aerobics*

WAKE UP: *8-oz glass of water*

MORNING SKIN CARE

DIET

BREAKFAST
· 2 slices turkey bacon
· 1 cup plain whole milk yogurt
· 1/2 cup strawberries
· 3 almonds
· Green or black tea or water
· 1 Total Skin & Body Vitamin Packet

LUNCH
· 4 to 6 ounces grilled chicken
· 1/2 cup vegetable barley soup
· Large green salad with sliced tomatoes
· 2-inch wedge of cantaloupe
· Green or black tea or water
· 1 Total Skin & Body Vitamin Packet

AFTERNOON SNACK
· 1 hard-boiled egg
· 2-inch wedge of cantaloupe
· 4 almonds
· Green or black tea or water

DINNER
· 6 ounces Scallops with Garlic and Parsley*
· Mediterranean Chopped Salad* with 1/2 cup chickpeas
· 1/2 cup cooked green beans
· Green or black tea or water

BEDTIME SNACK
· 2 slices turkey breast
· 4 green olives
· 1 apple

* Recipe available in *The Perricone Prescription: A Physician's 28-Day Program for Total Face and Body Rejuvenation.*

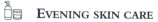 **EVENING SKIN CARE**

RECORD YOUR DAY'S ACTIVITIES, IMPRESSIONS, AND FEELINGS

TAKE A FEW MINUTES TO PRAY, MEDITATE, AND REFLECT

JOURNAL NOTES

THREE THINGS I APPRECIATED IN MY LIFE TODAY:
1. _____
2. _____
3. _____

SKIN

Face and Neck: _____ Fine Lines: _____

Dark Circles: _____ Puffiness: _____

Radiance: _____ Pore Size: _____

Firmness (jawline): _____

BODY

Weight: _____ Tone: _____

Energy: _____ Exercise: _____

MIND

Mood: _____ Stress: _____

Memory: _____ Problem-solving: _____

LIFESTYLE

Habits (coffee, alcohol, smoking): _____

Sleep (quality, number of hours): _____

Meditation/prayer: _____

OTHER NOTES, IMPRESSIONS, FEELINGS

_____

_____

_____

_____

> *Watch portion size—even good foods can cause an insulin response if we eat too much at one sitting.*

WEEK 6 / DAY 39   DATE: _____

EXERCISE FOR THE DAY: *weight training*

 WAKE UP: *8-oz glass of water*

MORNING SKIN CARE

DIET

BREAKFAST
- 4 ounces smoked salmon
- 3 ounces plain whole milk yogurt
- 1 tomato slice
- ¼ cantaloupe
- Green or black tea or water
- 1 Total Skin & Body Vitamin Packet

LUNCH
- 6 ounces canned crabmeat dressed with 1 tablespoon mayonnaise
- ½ cup lentil soup
- Large romaine lettuce salad dressed with olive oil and lemon to taste
- Green or black tea or water
- 1 Total Skin & Body Vitamin Packet

AFTERNOON SNACK
- 1 hard-boiled egg
- 4 cherry tomatoes
- 4 macadamia nuts
- Green or black tea or water

DINNER
- 6 ounces roast chicken breast (cook 8 ounces and save 2 ounces for tomorrow's lunch)
- ½ cup Manhattan Clam Chowder*
- ½ cup grilled eggplant topped with sliced tomato and 1 tablespoon grated Parmesan cheese
- Green or black tea or water

BEDTIME SNACK
- ½ cup cottage cheese
- ½ cup blueberries
- 4 hazelnuts

* Recipe available in *The Perricone Prescription: A Physician's 28-Day Program for Total Face and Body Rejuvenation.*

- **Evening skin care**
- **Record your day's activities, impressions, and feelings**
- **Take a few minutes to pray, meditate, and reflect**

JOURNAL NOTES

THREE THINGS I APPRECIATED IN MY LIFE TODAY:
1. _____
2. _____
3. _____

SKIN

Face and Neck: _____   Fine Lines: _____

Dark Circles: _____   Puffiness: _____

Radiance: _____   Pore Size: _____

Firmness (jawline): _____

BODY

Weight: _____   Tone: _____

Energy: _____   Exercise: _____

MIND

Mood: _____   Stress: _____

Memory: _____   Problem-solving: _____

LIFESTYLE

Habits (coffee, alcohol, smoking): _____

Sleep (quality, number of hours): _____

Meditation/prayer: _____

OTHER NOTES, IMPRESSIONS, FEELINGS

_____

_____

_____

_____

WEEK 6 / DAY 40   DATE: _____

EXERCISE FOR THE DAY: *aerobics (20 minutes' vigorous walking)*

WAKE UP: *8-oz glass of water*

MORNING SKIN CARE

DIET

BREAKFAST
· Scrambled eggs (3 egg whites and 1 yolk) with a little chopped onion
  and green bell peppers
· 2 slices turkey bacon
· 2-inch wedge cantaloupe
· Green or black tea or water
· 1 Total Skin & Body Vitamin Packet

LUNCH
· 3 to 5 ounces of chicken salad (made with 2 ounces chicken saved
  from last night's dinner, mixed with chopped red onion and celery,
  and dressed with 1 tablespoon olive oil and lemon juice) served on
  a bed of romaine lettuce
· Sliced tomatoes
· 1 cup Chicken-Vegetable Soup*
· Green or black tea or water
· 1 Total Skin & Body Vitamin Packet

AFTERNOON SNACK
· 1/2 cup plain whole milk yogurt
· 1/2 cup blueberries
· 1 teaspoon chopped almonds
· Green or black tea or water

DINNER
· 6 ounces grilled salmon
· Salad of romaine lettuce, avocado, and tomato, dressed with olive oil
  and lemon juice
· Grilled zucchini and mushroom kebabs
· Green or black tea or water

BEDTIME SNACK
· 2 ounces tuna salad (tuna mixed with onion, celery, pepper, and
  mustard or a touch or mayonnaise, if desired)
· 4 almonds
· 1 pear

* Recipe available in *The Perricone Prescription: A Physician's 28-Day Program for
Total Face and Body Rejuvenation.*

EVENING SKIN CARE

RECORD YOUR DAY'S ACTIVITIES, IMPRESSIONS, AND FEELINGS

TAKE A FEW MINUTES TO PRAY, MEDITATE, AND REFLECT

JOURNAL NOTES

THREE THINGS I APPRECIATED IN MY LIFE TODAY:

1. _____

2. _____

3. _____

SKIN

Face and Neck: _____   Fine Lines: _____

Dark Circles: _____   Puffiness: _____

Radiance: _____   Pore Size: _____

Firmness (jawline): _____

BODY

Weight: _____   Tone: _____

Energy: _____   Exercise: _____

MIND

Mood: _____   Stress: _____

Memory: _____   Problem-solving: _____

LIFESTYLE

Habits (coffee, alcohol, smoking): _____

Sleep (quality, number of hours): _____

Meditation/prayer: _____

OTHER NOTES, IMPRESSIONS, FEELINGS

_____

_____

_____

_____

> *Olive oil is one of **nature's greatest gifts** for preserving your health, beauty, and longevity.*

WEEK 6 / DAY 41   DATE: _____

 EXERCISE FOR THE DAY: *aerobics*

WAKE UP: *8-oz glass of water*

MORNING SKIN CARE

DIET

BREAKFAST
· 2 to 4 ounces smoked salmon
· $1/2$ cup plain whole milk yogurt
· 1 tablespoon chopped walnuts
· $1/2$ cup blueberries
· Green or black tea or water
· 1 Total Skin & Body Vitamin Packet

LUNCH
· Grilled Chicken Breast*
· Green salad topped with $1/2$ cup white or navy beans
· Steamed asparagus
· Green or black tea or water
· 1 Total Skin & Body Vitamin Packet

AFTERNOON SNACK
· 1 hard-boiled egg
· 2-inch wedge cantaloupe
· 4 macadamia nuts
· Green or black tea or water

DINNER
· 6 ounces grilled bluefin or albacore tuna steak
· $1/2$ cup grilled zucchini, eggplant, and red or green bell peppers lightly drizzled with olive oil and sprinkled with 1 tablespoon Parmesan cheese
· Tomato salsa (use fresh, if possible)
· Green or black tea or water

BEDTIME SNACK
· 2 slices turkey breast
· 4 green olives
· 4 cherry tomatoes

* Recipe available in *The Perricone Prescription: A Physician's 28-Day Program for Total Face and Body Rejuvenation.*

Evening skin care

Record your day's activities, impressions, and feelings

Take a few minutes to pray, meditate, and reflect

JOURNAL NOTES

THREE THINGS I APPRECIATED IN MY LIFE TODAY:
1. _____
2. _____
3. _____

SKIN

Face and Neck: _____   Fine Lines: _____

Dark Circles: _____   Puffiness: _____

Radiance: _____   Pore Size: _____

Firmness (jawline): _____

BODY

Weight: _____   Tone: _____

Energy: _____   Exercise: _____

MIND

Mood: _____   Stress: _____

Memory: _____   Problem-solving: _____

LIFESTYLE

Habits (coffee, alcohol, smoking): _____

Sleep (quality, number of hours): _____

Meditation/prayer: _____

OTHER NOTES, IMPRESSIONS, FEELINGS

_____
_____
_____
_____

> *A dehydrated body provokes the development of aging. Even mild dehydration can result in the gain of* **one pound of fat every six months.**

WEEK 6 / DAY 42   DATE: _____

EXERCISE FOR THE DAY: *relaxation (you've* **REALLY** *earned it!)*

WAKE UP: *8-oz glass of water*

MORNING SKIN CARE

DIET

BREAKFAST
- Omelet made with 3 egg whites, 1 yolk, and a few sliced fresh mushrooms
- $1/2$ cup slow-cooked oatmeal
- 1 teaspoon chopped almonds
- 2-inch wedge cantaloupe
- Green or black tea or water
- 1 Total Skin & Body Vitamin Packet

LUNCH
- 3 to 4 ounces water-packed tuna
- Romaine lettuce salad made with $1/2$ cup white beans, $1/4$ cup crumbled feta cheese, 4 cherry tomatoes, and sliced red onion, dressed with olive oil and lemon juice
- Green or black tea or water
- 1 Total Skin & Body Vitamin Packet

AFTERNOON SNACK
- 1 slice turkey breast
- 4 hazelnuts
- 2-inch wedge cantaloupe
- Green or black tea or water

DINNER
- 4 large shrimp, grilled, broiled, or baked on skewers with mushrooms, onions, and cherry tomatoes
- $1/2$ cup Cuban Black Bean Soup*
- Romaine lettuce salad dressed with olive oil and lemon juice
- Green or black tea or water

BEDTIME SNACK
- 2 slices turkey breast
- 4 green olives
- 4 cherry tomatoes

* Recipe available in *The Perricone Prescription: A Physician's 28-Day Program for Total Face and Body Rejuvenation.*

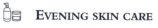 **EVENING SKIN CARE**

📖 **RECORD YOUR DAY'S ACTIVITIES, IMPRESSIONS, AND FEELINGS**

☁ **TAKE A FEW MINUTES TO PRAY, MEDITATE, AND REFLECT**

JOURNAL NOTES

THREE THINGS I APPRECIATED IN MY LIFE TODAY:

1. _____
2. _____
3. _____

SKIN

Face and Neck: _____   Fine Lines: _____

Dark Circles: _____   Puffiness: _____

Radiance: _____   Pore Size: _____

Firmness (jawline): _____

BODY

Weight: _____   Tone: _____

Energy: _____   Exercise: _____

MIND

Mood: _____   Stress: _____

Memory: _____   Problem-solving: _____

LIFESTYLE

Habits (coffee, alcohol, smoking): _____

Sleep (quality, number of hours): _____

Meditation/prayer: _____

OTHER NOTES, IMPRESSIONS, FEELINGS

_____
_____
_____
_____

> *Drinking hard liquor causes inflammatory problems in the body. In short: wine is fine… but **forget the martini**.*

WEEK 7 / DAY 43   DATE: _____

EXERCISE FOR THE DAY: *aerobics (20 minutes' vigorous walking)*

WAKE UP: *8-oz glass of water*

MORNING SKIN CARE

DIET

BREAKFAST
- 2 ounces smoked salmon
- 6 ounces plain whole milk yogurt
- 2-inch wedge cantaloupe
- Green or black tea or water
- 1 Total Skin & Body Vitamin Packet

LUNCH
- 1 6-ounce can shrimp (drained) mixed with 1 tablespoon olive oil and juice of $1/2$ lemon, served inside $1/2$ avocado
- $1/2$ cup cherries
- Green or black tea or water
- 1 Total Skin & Body Vitamin Packet

AFTERNOON SNACK
- 2 ounces sliced turkey or chicken breast
- 4 almonds
- 4 cherry tomatoes
- Green or black tea or water

DINNER
- 4 to 6 ounces baked scrod fillets
- $1/2$ cup steamed broccoli or spinach
- Tossed green salad dressed with olive oil and lemon juice
- Green or black tea or water

BEDTIME SNACK
- 1 hard-boiled egg
- 3 celery sticks
- 3 green olives

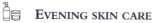 **Evening skin care**

📖 **Record your day's activities, impressions, and feelings**

☁️ **Take a few minutes to pray, meditate, and reflect**

Journal Notes

> **THREE THINGS I APPRECIATED IN MY LIFE TODAY:**
> 1. _____
> 2. _____
> 3. _____

SKIN

Face and Neck: _____   Fine Lines: _____

Dark Circles: _____   Puffiness: _____

Radiance: _____   Pore Size: _____

Firmness (jawline): _____

BODY

Weight: _____   Tone: _____

Energy: _____   Exercise: _____

MIND

Mood: _____   Stress: _____

Memory: _____   Problem-solving: _____

LIFESTYLE

Habits (coffee, alcohol, smoking): _____

Sleep (quality, number of hours): _____

Meditation/prayer: _____

OTHER NOTES, IMPRESSIONS, FEELINGS

_____

_____

_____

_____

> *A **good night's sleep** can help you awake refreshed, looking radiant and youthful. And, after a good night's sleep, doesn't the world look better, too?*

WEEK 7 / DAY 44   DATE: _____

EXERCISE FOR THE DAY: *weight training*

 WAKE UP: *8-oz glass of water*

MORNING SKIN CARE

DIET

BREAKFAST
- Omelet made with 2 eggs, fresh herbs, and a few sliced fresh mushrooms
- $1/2$ cup slow-cooked oatmeal
- 3 hazelnuts
- $1/2$ cup blueberries
- Green or black tea or water
- 1 Total Skin & Body Vitamin Packet

LUNCH
- 3 to 6 ounces canned salmon mixed with 1 teaspoon mayonnaise
- Green salad with sliced tomatoes, cucumbers, and 2 tablespoons chickpeas; dressed with olive oil and lemon juice
- 2-inch wedge honeydew melon
- Green or black tea or water
- 1 Total Skin & Body Vitamin Packet

AFTERNOON SNACK
- 6 ounces plain whole milk yogurt
- 3 hazelnuts
- $1/4$ cup fresh berries
- Green or black tea or water

DINNER
- 4 to 6 ounces baked or grilled trout
- Three-bean salad made with $1/2$ cup lentils, $1/2$ cup green beans, and $1/2$ cup chickpeas; dressed with olive oil and lemon juice
- $1/2$ cup steamed and mashed turnip
- 1 pear
- Green or black tea or water

BEDTIME SNACK
- 2 ounces sliced roast turkey breast
- 4 almonds
- 3 radishes

□▤ EVENING SKIN CARE

▤ RECORD YOUR DAY'S ACTIVITIES, IMPRESSIONS, AND FEELINGS

☁ TAKE A FEW MINUTES TO PRAY, MEDITATE, AND REFLECT

JOURNAL NOTES

THREE THINGS I APPRECIATED IN MY LIFE TODAY:

1. _____

2. _____

3. _____

SKIN

Face and Neck: _____   Fine Lines: _____

Dark Circles: _____   Puffiness: _____

Radiance: _____   Pore Size: _____

Firmness (jawline): _____

BODY

Weight: _____   Tone: _____

Energy: _____   Exercise: _____

MIND

Mood: _____   Stress: _____

Memory: _____   Problem-solving: _____

LIFESTYLE

Habits (coffee, alcohol, smoking): _____

Sleep (quality, number of hours): _____

Meditation/prayer: _____

OTHER NOTES, IMPRESSIONS, FEELINGS

_____

_____

_____

_____

> *Extra virgin olive oil increases the skin's ability to*
> **maintain moisture.**

WEEK 7 / DAY 45 DATE: _____

 EXERCISE FOR THE DAY: *aerobics*

WAKE UP: *8-oz glass of water*

MORNING SKIN CARE

DIET

BREAKFAST
- 2 slices turkey bacon
- 1/2 cup slow-cooked oatmeal
- 3 hazelnuts
- 1/2 grapefruit
- Green or black tea or water
- 1 Total Skin & Body Vitamin Packet

LUNCH
- 3- to 4-ounce can tuna or sardines
- 1 cup sliced tomatoes and cucumbers
- 1/2 cup lentil soup
- Green or black tea or water
- 1 Total Skin & Body Vitamin Packet

AFTERNOON SNACK
- 6 ounces plain whole milk yogurt
- 4 chopped almonds
- 1 small apple
- Green or black tea or water

DINNER
- 4 to 6 ounces broiled fillet of salmon
- 1 cup steamed asparagus
- Romaine lettuce salad with 1/4 cup chickpeas; dressed with olive oil and lemon juice
- Green or black tea or water

BEDTIME SNACK
- 2 ounces sliced turkey or chicken breast
- 4 black olives
- 1 kiwi fruit

EVENING SKIN CARE

RECORD YOUR DAY'S ACTIVITIES, IMPRESSIONS, AND FEELINGS

TAKE A FEW MINUTES TO PRAY, MEDITATE, AND REFLECT

JOURNAL NOTES

THREE THINGS I APPRECIATED IN MY LIFE TODAY:
1. _____
2. _____
3. _____

SKIN

Face and Neck: _____   Fine Lines: _____

Dark Circles: _____   Puffiness: _____

Radiance: _____   Pore Size: _____

Firmness (jawline): _____

BODY

Weight: _____   Tone: _____

Energy: _____   Exercise: _____

MIND

Mood: _____   Stress: _____

Memory: _____   Problem-solving: _____

LIFESTYLE

Habits (coffee, alcohol, smoking): _____

Sleep (quality, number of hours): _____

Meditation/prayer: _____

OTHER NOTES, IMPRESSIONS, FEELINGS

_____

_____

_____

_____

> ***Brain function** is intimately tied to our essential fatty acid intake.*

WEEK 7 / DAY 46   DATE: _____

EXERCISE FOR THE DAY: *aerobics (20 minutes' vigorous walking)*

WAKE UP: *8-oz glass of water*

MORNING SKIN CARE

DIET

BREAKFAST
· 2 links turkey sausage
· 1 soft-boiled egg
· 1/2 cup slow-cooked oatmeal
· 2-inch wedge cantaloupe
· Green or black tea or water
· 1 Total Skin & Body Vitamin Packet

LUNCH
· 4 ounces chicken salad (diced chicken breast mixed with fresh dill, chopped red onion, chopped celery; dressed with olive oil and lemon juice) served on a bed of romaine lettuce
· 4 hazelnuts
· 1 apple
· Green or black tea or water
· 1 Total Skin & Body Vitamin Packet

AFTERNOON SNACK
· 6 ounces plain whole milk yogurt
· 4 almonds
· 1/4 cup fresh cherries
· Green or black tea or water

DINNER
· 6 ounces broiled fillet of sole, cod, or scrod. (Make 8 ounces and save 2 ounces for tomorrow's bedtime snack.)
· 1 cup steamed spinach
· Romaine lettuce salad with 1/4 cup chickpeas; dressed with olive oil, minced garlic, and lemon juice
· 1/2 cup mixed fresh berries
· Green or black tea or water

BEDTIME SNACK
· 3-ounce can tuna
· 4 macadamia nuts
· 1 pear

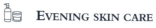

Evening skin care

Record your day's activities, impressions, and feelings

Take a few minutes to pray, meditate, and reflect

Journal Notes

> **THREE THINGS I APPRECIATED IN MY LIFE TODAY:**
> 1. _____
> 2. _____
> 3. _____

SKIN

Face and Neck: _____ Fine Lines: _____

Dark Circles: _____ Puffiness: _____

Radiance: _____ Pore Size: _____

Firmness (jawline): _____

BODY

Weight: _____ Tone: _____

Energy: _____ Exercise: _____

MIND

Mood: _____ Stress: _____

Memory: _____ Problem-solving: _____

LIFESTYLE

Habits (coffee, alcohol, smoking): _____

Sleep (quality, number of hours): _____

Meditation/prayer: _____

OTHER NOTES, IMPRESSIONS, FEELINGS

_____

_____

_____

_____

> *From asparagus to zucchini,* **fresh fruits and vegetables** *are nature's storehouse of antioxidants.*

WEEK 7 / DAY 47   DATE: _____

✚ **EXERCISE FOR THE DAY:** *aerobics (20 minutes' vigorous walking)*

💧 **WAKE UP:** *8-oz glass of water*

🧴 **MORNING SKIN CARE**

✗ **DIET**

BREAKFAST
- 3 strips turkey bacon
- $1/2$ cup slow-cooked oatmeal
- 4 hazelnuts
- 2-inch wedge cantaloupe
- Green or black tea or water
- 1 Total Skin & Body Vitamin Packet

LUNCH
- 4 ounces salmon salad (finely cubed salmon fillet or canned salmon dressed with lemon juice, olive oil, and fresh dill) served on a bed of romaine lettuce
- $1/2$ cup lentil soup
- 1 kiwi fruit
- Green or black tea or water
- 1 Total Skin & Body Vitamin Packet

AFTERNOON SNACK
- 2 slices turkey breast
- $1/4$ cup fresh strawberries
- 4 hazelnuts
- Green or black tea or water

DINNER
- 6 ounces baked chicken breast (skin removed)
- $1/2$ cup sautéed zucchini or summer squash topped with 4 chopped almonds
- $1/2$ cup Three Bean Salad*
- 2-inch wedge honeydew melon
- Green or black tea or water

BEDTIME SNACK
- 2 ounces cold fillet of sole, cod, or scrod
- 3 macadamia nuts
- 3 cherry tomatoes

* Recipe available in *The Perricone Prescription: A Physician's 28-Day Program for Total Face and Body Rejuvenation.*

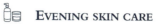

EVENING SKIN CARE

RECORD YOUR DAY'S ACTIVITIES, IMPRESSIONS, AND FEELINGS

TAKE A FEW MINUTES TO PRAY, MEDITATE, AND REFLECT

JOURNAL NOTES

THREE THINGS I APPRECIATED IN MY LIFE TODAY:
1. _____
2. _____
3. _____

SKIN

Face and Neck: _____   Fine Lines: _____

Dark Circles: _____   Puffiness: _____

Radiance: _____   Pore Size: _____

Firmness (jawline): _____

BODY

Weight: _____   Tone: _____

Energy: _____   Exercise: _____

MIND

Mood: _____   Stress: _____

Memory: _____   Problem-solving: _____

LIFESTYLE

Habits (coffee, alcohol, smoking): _____

Sleep (quality, number of hours): _____

Meditation/prayer: _____

OTHER NOTES, IMPRESSIONS, FEELINGS

_____
_____
_____
_____

> *Exercise is vital for your health. Studies have shown that **exercise benefits the skin** in much the same way it improves bone and muscle quality.*

WEEK 7 / DAY 48   DATE: _____

 EXERCISE FOR THE DAY: *weight training*

WAKE UP: *8-oz glass of water*

MORNING SKIN CARE

DIET

BREAKFAST
· Omelet made with 2 eggs, 1 ounce crumbled feta cheese, and ½ teaspoon fresh dill
· 2 ounces smoked salmon
· ½ cup blueberries
· Green or black tea or water
· 1 Total Skin & Body Vitamin Packet

LUNCH
· 4 to 6 ounces broiled turkey burger (no bun)
· 1 cup salad made with cherry tomatoes, sliced cucumbers, and chopped red onion; dressed with olive oil and lemon juice
· 1 apple
· Green or black tea or water
· 1 Total Skin & Body Vitamin Packet

AFTERNOON SNACK
· 6 ounces plain whole milk yogurt
· ¼ cup sliced fresh strawberries
· Green or black tea or water

DINNER
· 4 to 6 ounces baked or grilled halibut or sea bass
· 1 cup steamed asparagus
· Romaine lettuce salad with ¼ cup chickpeas, dressed with olive oil and lemon juice
· 2-inch wedge cantaloupe
· Green or black tea or water

BEDTIME SNACK
· 2 slices roast turkey or chicken breast
· 4 macadamia nuts
· ¼ cup fresh cherries

* Recipe available in *The Perricone Prescription: A Physician's 28-Day Program for Total Face and Body Rejuvenation.*

Evening skin care

Record your day's activities, impressions, and feelings

Take a few minutes to pray, meditate, and reflect

JOURNAL NOTES

THREE THINGS I APPRECIATED IN MY LIFE TODAY:

1. _____
2. _____
3. _____

SKIN

Face and Neck: _____   Fine Lines: _____

Dark Circles: _____   Puffiness: _____

Radiance: _____   Pore Size: _____

Firmness (jawline): _____

BODY

Weight: _____   Tone: _____

Energy: _____   Exercise: _____

MIND

Mood: _____   Stress: _____

Memory: _____   Problem-solving: _____

LIFESTYLE

Habits (coffee, alcohol, smoking): _____

Sleep (quality, number of hours): _____

Meditation/prayer: _____

OTHER NOTES, IMPRESSIONS, FEELINGS

_____

_____

_____

_____

> *All skin tones are vulnerable to damage from the sun's ultraviolet rays.* **Applying sunscreen** *at the start of your day should be as automatic as combing your hair.*

WEEK 7 / DAY 49   DATE: _____

EXERCISE FOR THE DAY: *relaxation*

WAKE UP: *8-oz glass of water*

 MORNING SKIN CARE

DIET

BREAKFAST
- 3 ounces broiled salmon
- $1/2$ cup slow-cooked oatmeal
- 2-inch wedge cantaloupe
- Green or black tea or water
- 1 Total Skin & Body Vitamin Packet

LUNCH
- 6-ounce can of tuna or sardines
- Greek salad with romaine lettuce, 3 black olives, 1 ounce feta cheese, $1/2$ sliced cucumber, 4 cherry tomatoes; dress with olive oil, lemon juice, dash of oregano; toss
- $1/2$ cup mixed fresh berries
- Green or black tea or water
- 1 Total Skin & Body Vitamin Packet

AFTERNOON SNACK
- $1/2$ cup plain cottage cheese
- 4 hazelnuts
- 1 apple
- Green or black tea or water

DINNER
- Chicken Stir Fry (6 ounces chicken breast chopped into 1-inch strips; $1/4$ cup each sliced mushrooms, chopped onions, water chestnuts, chopped almonds, bamboo shoots, bok choy or celery, and mung bean sprouts; toss together and stir fry in olive oil)
- Romaine lettuce salad dressed with olive oil and lemon juice
- 2-inch wedge cantaloupe
- Green or black tea or water

BEDTIME SNACK
- 2 slices turkey breast
- 3 olives
- 1 pear

- **Evening skin care**
- **Record your day's activities, impressions, and feelings**
- **Take a few minutes to pray, meditate, and reflect**

Journal Notes

THREE THINGS I APPRECIATED IN MY LIFE TODAY:
1. _____
2. _____
3. _____

SKIN

Face and Neck: _____   Fine Lines: _____

Dark Circles: _____   Puffiness: _____

Radiance: _____   Pore Size: _____

Firmness (jawline): _____

BODY

Weight: _____   Tone: _____

Energy: _____   Exercise: _____

MIND

Mood: _____   Stress: _____

Memory: _____   Problem-solving: _____

LIFESTYLE

Habits (coffee, alcohol, smoking): _____

Sleep (quality, number of hours): _____

Meditation/prayer: _____

OTHER NOTES, IMPRESSIONS, FEELINGS

_____

_____

_____

_____

> *Food is much more than just a life-giving and life-sustaining substance—it is our **single most powerful** anti-aging tool.*

WEEK 8 / DAY 50   DATE: _____

EXERCISE FOR THE DAY: *aerobics (20 minutes' vigorous walking)*

WAKE UP: *8-oz glass of water*

MORNING SKIN CARE

DIET

BREAKFAST
- 2 links turkey sausage
- 1 soft-boiled egg
- $1/2$ grapefruit
- Green or black tea or water
- 1 Total Skin & Body Vitamin Packet

LUNCH
- 6-ounce canned crabmeat mixed with 1 teaspoon mayonnaise and 1 chopped celery stalk
- $1/2$ cup lentil soup
- 1 apple
- Green or black tea or water
- 1 Total Skin & Body Vitamin Packet

AFTERNOON SNACK
- 2 ounces smoked salmon
- 2-inch wedge cantaloupe
- Green or black tea or water

DINNER
- 6 ounces scallops sautéed with minced garlic in olive oil. (Cook 8 ounces and save 2 ounces for tomorrow's lunch.)
- $1/2$ cup steamed broccoli
- $1/4$ cup fresh cherries
- Green or black tea or water

BEDTIME SNACK
- 6 ounces plain whole milk yogurt
- 4 hazelnuts
- $1/4$ cup blueberries

EVENING SKIN CARE

RECORD YOUR DAY'S ACTIVITIES, IMPRESSIONS, AND FEELINGS

TAKE A FEW MINUTES TO PRAY, MEDITATE, AND REFLECT

JOURNAL NOTES

THREE THINGS I APPRECIATED IN MY LIFE TODAY:
1. _____
2. _____
3. _____

SKIN

Face and Neck: _____   Fine Lines: _____

Dark Circles: _____   Puffiness: _____

Radiance: _____   Pore Size: _____

Firmness (jawline): _____

BODY

Weight: _____   Tone: _____

Energy: _____   Exercise: _____

MIND

Mood: _____   Stress: _____

Memory: _____   Problem-solving: _____

LIFESTYLE

Habits (coffee, alcohol, smoking): _____

Sleep (quality, number of hours): _____

Meditation/prayer: _____

OTHER NOTES, IMPRESSIONS, FEELINGS

_____

_____

_____

_____

WEEK 8 / DAY 51　　　　DATE: _____

EXERCISE FOR THE DAY: *weight training*

WAKE UP: *8-oz glass of water*

MORNING SKIN CARE

DIET

BREAKFAST
· Vegetable omelet made with 2 eggs and $\frac{1}{4}$ cup each chopped onions,
  sliced mushrooms, and chopped green pepper
· $\frac{1}{2}$ cup slow-cooked oatmeal
· 3 hazelnuts
· $\frac{1}{2}$ grapefruit
· Green or black tea or water
· 1 Total Skin & Body Vitamin Packet

LUNCH
· Scallop salad made with 2 ounces scallops (from previous night's
  dinner), chopped red onion, 3 chopped black olives and fresh dill,
  dressed with olive oil and lemon juice
· 2-inch wedge honeydew melon
· Green or black tea or water
· 1 Total Skin & Body Vitamin Packet

AFTERNOON SNACK
· 6 ounces plain whole milk yogurt
· $\frac{1}{4}$ cup fresh blueberries, blackberries, or raspberries
· 3 macadamia nuts
· Green or black tea or water

DINNER
· 6 ounces grilled salmon
· $\frac{1}{2}$ cup lentil soup
· Romaine lettuce salad dressed with olive oil and lemon juice
· $\frac{1}{2}$ cup fresh cherries
· Green or black tea or water

BEDTIME SNACK
· $\frac{1}{2}$ cup plain cottage cheese
· 3 strawberries
· 4 hazelnuts

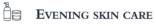

EVENING SKIN CARE

RECORD YOUR DAY'S ACTIVITIES, IMPRESSIONS, AND FEELINGS

TAKE A FEW MINUTES TO PRAY, MEDITATE, AND REFLECT

JOURNAL NOTES

THREE THINGS I APPRECIATED IN MY LIFE TODAY:

1. _____

2. _____

3. _____

SKIN

Face and Neck: _____   Fine Lines: _____

Dark Circles: _____   Puffiness: _____

Radiance: _____   Pore Size: _____

Firmness (jawline): _____

BODY

Weight: _____   Tone: _____

Energy: _____   Exercise: _____

MIND

Mood: _____   Stress: _____

Memory: _____   Problem-solving: _____

LIFESTYLE

Habits (coffee, alcohol, smoking): _____

Sleep (quality, number of hours): _____

Meditation/prayer: _____

OTHER NOTES, IMPRESSIONS, FEELINGS

_____

_____

_____

_____

WEEK 8 / DAY 52   DATE: _____

 EXERCISE FOR THE DAY: *aerobics (20 minutes' vigorous walking)*

WAKE UP: *8-oz glass of water*

MORNING SKIN CARE

DIET

BREAKFAST
- 2 links turkey sausage
- 1 poached egg
- 3 almonds
- 2-inch wedge cantaloupe
- Green or black tea or water
- 1 Total Skin & Body Vitamin Packet

LUNCH
- 4 to 6 ounces grilled chicken breast
- Romaine lettuce salad with sliced tomatoes and $1/4$ cup chickpeas; dressed with olive oil and lemon juice
- $1/2$ cup fresh cherries
- Green or black tea or water
- 1 Total Skin & Body Vitamin Packet

AFTERNOON SNACK
- 6 ounces plain whole milk yogurt
- 4 hazelnuts
- 1 kiwi fruit
- Green or black tea or water

DINNER
- 6 ounces broiled trout
- Mixed three-leaf salad (arugula, radicchio, and endive) dressed with olive oil and lemon juice
- $1/2$ cup green beans garnished with chopped almonds
- Green or black tea or water

BEDTIME SNACK
- 2 slices chicken or turkey breast
- 4 macadamia nuts
- 1 small pear

EVENING SKIN CARE

RECORD YOUR DAY'S ACTIVITIES, IMPRESSIONS, AND FEELINGS

TAKE A FEW MINUTES TO PRAY, MEDITATE, AND REFLECT

JOURNAL NOTES

THREE THINGS I APPRECIATED IN MY LIFE TODAY:
1. _____
2. _____
3. _____

SKIN

Face and Neck: _____   Fine Lines: _____

Dark Circles: _____   Puffiness: _____

Radiance: _____   Pore Size: _____

Firmness (jawline): _____

BODY

Weight: _____   Tone: _____

Energy: _____   Exercise: _____

MIND

Mood: _____   Stress: _____

Memory: _____   Problem-solving: _____

LIFESTYLE

Habits (coffee, alcohol, smoking): _____

Sleep (quality, number of hours): _____

Meditation/prayer: _____

OTHER NOTES, IMPRESSIONS, FEELINGS

_____
_____
_____
_____

> *A diet rich in **high quality protein** will firm up the face and body in a matter of weeks.*

WEEK 8 / DAY 53   DATE: _____

EXERCISE FOR THE DAY: *weight training*

 WAKE UP: *8-oz glass of water*

MORNING SKIN CARE

DIET

BREAKFAST
· 4 ounces smoked salmon
· 1 slice tomato
· 1/2 grapefruit
· Green or black tea or water
· 1 Total Skin & Body Vitamin Packet

LUNCH
· Crabmeat salad (1 6-ounce can of crabmeat mixed with 1 chopped scallion, 1 chopped celery rib, 1/4 cup plain yogurt and juice of 1/2 lemon) served inside 1/2 avocado
· 1/2 cup lentil soup
· Green or black tea or water
· 1 Total Skin & Body Vitamin Packet

AFTERNOON SNACK
· 1 hard-boiled egg
· 4 cherry tomatoes
· 4 macadamia nuts
· Green or black tea or water

DINNER
· 6 ounces baked turkey breast.
· 1 small eggplant, sliced and grilled, topped with sliced tomato and 1 tablespoon grated Parmesan cheese
· 1 apple
· Green or black tea or water

BEDTIME SNACK
· 6 ounces plain whole milk yogurt
· 4 hazelnuts
· 1/4 cup blueberries

☐☐ **E**VENING SKIN CARE

📖 **R**ECORD YOUR DAY'S ACTIVITIES, IMPRESSIONS, AND FEELINGS

☁ **T**AKE A FEW MINUTES TO PRAY, MEDITATE, AND REFLECT

JOURNAL NOTES

THREE THINGS I APPRECIATED IN MY LIFE TODAY:
1. _____
2. _____
3. _____

SKIN

Face and Neck: _____   Fine Lines: _____

Dark Circles: _____   Puffiness: _____

Radiance: _____   Pore Size: _____

Firmness (jawline): _____

BODY

Weight: _____   Tone: _____

Energy: _____   Exercise: _____

MIND

Mood: _____   Stress: _____

Memory: _____   Problem-solving: _____

LIFESTYLE

Habits (coffee, alcohol, smoking): _____

Sleep (quality, number of hours): _____

Meditation/prayer: _____

OTHER NOTES, IMPRESSIONS, FEELINGS

_____

_____

_____

_____

WEEK 8 / DAY 54   DATE: _____

EXERCISE FOR THE DAY: *aerobics (20 minutes' vigorous walking)*

WAKE UP: *8-oz glass of water*

MORNING SKIN CARE

DIET

BREAKFAST
- 2 slices turkey bacon
- 2 soft-boiled eggs
- 2-inch wedge cantaloupe
- Green or black tea or water
- 1 Total Skin & Body Vitamin Packet

LUNCH
- 3 to 5 ounces chicken salad (mix 2 ounces chicken saved from last night's dinner with 1 teaspoon each chopped red onion and celery, 4 chopped hazelnuts, and 1 tablespoon olive oil and lemon juice) served on a bed of romaine lettuce
- 1 pear
- Green or black tea or water
- 1 Total Skin & Body Vitamin Packet

AFTERNOON SNACK
- 6 ounces plain whole milk yogurt
- 1/4 cup fresh cherries
- 4 hazelnuts
- Green or black tea or water

DINNER
- 6 ounces grilled salmon
- Salad of romaine lettuce, avocado, and tomato, dressed with olive oil and lemon juice
- 1 cup steamed asparagus
- Green or black tea or water

BEDTIME SNACK
- 2 ounces tuna
- 4 green or black olives
- 1/4 cup blueberries

- EVENING SKIN CARE

- RECORD YOUR DAY'S ACTIVITIES, IMPRESSIONS, AND FEELINGS

- TAKE A FEW MINUTES TO PRAY, MEDITATE, AND REFLECT

JOURNAL NOTES

THREE THINGS I APPRECIATED IN MY LIFE TODAY:

1. _____
2. _____
3. _____

SKIN

Face and Neck: _____   Fine Lines: _____

Dark Circles: _____   Puffiness: _____

Radiance: _____   Pore Size: _____

Firmness (jawline): _____

BODY

Weight: _____   Tone: _____

Energy: _____   Exercise: _____

MIND

Mood: _____   Stress: _____

Memory: _____   Problem-solving: _____

LIFESTYLE

Habits (coffee, alcohol, smoking): _____

Sleep (quality, number of hours): _____

Meditation/prayer: _____

OTHER NOTES, IMPRESSIONS, FEELINGS

_____

_____

_____

_____

> *Researchers in Boston found patients with manic-depressive disorder who had not responded to conventional treatment **improved dramatically** when given a daily four-ounce serving of salmon.*

WEEK 8 / DAY 55   DATE: _____

EXERCISE FOR THE DAY: *aerobics*

WAKE UP: *8-oz glass of water*

MORNING SKIN CARE

DIET

BREAKFAST
- 2 to 4 ounces smoked salmon
- 6 ounces plain whole milk yogurt
- 4 chopped walnuts
- $^1/_2$ grapefruit
- Green or black tea or water
- 1 Total Skin & Body Vitamin Packet

LUNCH
- 6 ounces grilled turkey burger topped with romaine lettuce, sliced tomato, alfalfa sprouts, and red onion (no bun)
- $^1/_2$ cup lentil soup
- 2-inch wedge honeydew melon
- Green or black tea or water
- 1 Total Skin & Body Vitamin Packet

AFTERNOON SNACK
- 2 ounces sliced chicken breast
- 2-inch wedge cantaloupe
- 4 macadamia nuts
- Green or black tea or water

DINNER
- 6 ounces grilled bluefin or albacore tuna steak
- 1 cup steamed spinach
- Romaine lettuce salad tossed with olive oil and lemon juice
- $^1/_4$ cup mixed fresh berries
- Green or black tea or water

BEDTIME SNACK
- 2 slices turkey breast
- 4 green olives
- 4 cherry tomatoes

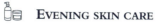 **EVENING SKIN CARE**

📖 **RECORD YOUR DAY'S ACTIVITIES, IMPRESSIONS, AND FEELINGS**

☁ **TAKE A FEW MINUTES TO PRAY, MEDITATE, AND REFLECT**

JOURNAL NOTES

THREE THINGS I APPRECIATED IN MY LIFE TODAY:
1. _____
2. _____
3. _____

SKIN

Face and Neck: _____   Fine Lines: _____

Dark Circles: _____   Puffiness: _____

Radiance: _____   Pore Size: _____

Firmness (jawline): _____

BODY

Weight: _____   Tone: _____

Energy: _____   Exercise: _____

MIND

Mood: _____   Stress: _____

Memory: _____   Problem-solving: _____

LIFESTYLE

Habits (coffee, alcohol, smoking): _____

Sleep (quality, number of hours): _____

Meditation/prayer: _____

OTHER NOTES, IMPRESSIONS, FEELINGS

_____

_____

_____

_____

> *Once you accept that your **everyday lifestyle choices**
> affect the way you age, you are on your way toward
> restoring youthful looks and vigor.*

WEEK 8 / DAY 56   DATE: _____

 EXERCISE FOR THE DAY: *relaxation*

WAKE UP: *8-oz glass of water*

MORNING SKIN CARE

DIET

BREAKFAST
- 2 ounces smoked salmon
- $1/2$ cup slow-cooked oatmeal
- 2-inch wedge cantaloupe
- Green or black tea or water
- 1 Total Skin & Body Vitamin Packet

LUNCH
- 3 to 4 ounces tuna tossed with $1/2$ cup white beans, 4 cherry tomatoes, and sliced red onion; dress with olive oil and lemon juice and serve on a bed of romaine lettuce
- 1 apple
- Green or black tea or water
- 1 Total Skin & Body Vitamin Packet

AFTERNOON SNACK
- 6 ounces plain whole milk yogurt
- 4 hazelnuts
- $1/2$ grapefruit
- Green or black tea or water

DINNER
- 4 large shrimp, brushed with olive oil and baked
- Salad of romaine lettuce, $1/4$ cup chickpeas, chopped celery, sliced tomato, and sliced avocado; dress with oil and lemon juice
- $1/4$ cup mixed fresh berries
- Green or black tea or water

BEDTIME SNACK
- $1/2$ cup cottage cheese
- 4 hazelnuts
- 1 pear

EVENING SKIN CARE

RECORD YOUR DAY'S ACTIVITIES, IMPRESSIONS, AND FEELINGS

TAKE A FEW MINUTES TO PRAY, MEDITATE, AND REFLECT

JOURNAL NOTES

THREE THINGS I APPRECIATED IN MY LIFE TODAY:

1. _____

2. _____

3. _____

SKIN

Face and Neck: _____ Fine Lines: _____

Dark Circles: _____ Puffiness: _____

Radiance: _____ Pore Size: _____

Firmness (jawline): _____

BODY

Weight: _____ Tone: _____

Energy: _____ Exercise: _____

MIND

Mood: _____ Stress: _____

Memory: _____ Problem-solving: _____

LIFESTYLE

Habits (coffee, alcohol, smoking): _____

Sleep (quality, number of hours): _____

Meditation/prayer: _____

OTHER NOTES, IMPRESSIONS, FEELINGS

_____

_____

_____

_____

> *Planning and preparation* will keep you out of the kitchen and away from temptation.

WEEK 9 / DAY 57   DATE: _____

EXERCISE FOR THE DAY: *aerobics*

WAKE UP: *8-oz glass of water*

MORNING SKIN CARE

DIET

BREAKFAST
- 3 to 4 ounces smoked Nova Scotia salmon
- $1/2$ cup slow-cooked oatmeal with 2 tablespoons blueberries
- 1 teaspoon slivered almonds
- Green or black tea or water
- 1 Total Skin & Body Vitamin Packet

LUNCH
- 4- to 6-ounce broiled turkey burger (no bun)
- Lettuce and tomato
- $1/2$ cup Three-Bean Salad*
- Green or black tea or water
- 1 Total Skin & Body Vitamin Packet

AFTERNOON SNACK
- 2 ounces sliced turkey or chicken breast
- 4 hazelnuts
- 4 celery sticks
- Green or black tea or water

DINNER
- 4 to 6 ounces broiled salmon
- 1 cup lentil soup
- Tossed green salad dressed with olive oil and lemon juice
- $1/2$ cup steamed spinach
- Green or black tea or water

BEDTIME SNACK
- 1 hard-boiled egg
- 3 celery sticks
- 3 red bell pepper strips
- 3 green olives

* Recipe available in *The Perricone Prescription: A Physician's 28-Day Program for Total Face and Body Rejuvenation.*

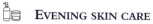 **EVENING SKIN CARE**

📖 **RECORD YOUR DAY'S ACTIVITIES, IMPRESSIONS, AND FEELINGS**

☁ **TAKE A FEW MINUTES TO PRAY, MEDITATE, AND REFLECT**

JOURNAL NOTES

THREE THINGS I APPRECIATED IN MY LIFE TODAY:
1. _____
2. _____
3. _____

SKIN

Face and Neck: _____   Fine Lines: _____

Dark Circles: _____   Puffiness: _____

Radiance: _____   Pore Size: _____

Firmness (jawline): _____

BODY

Weight: _____   Tone: _____

Energy: _____   Exercise: _____

MIND

Mood: _____   Stress: _____

Memory: _____   Problem-solving: _____

LIFESTYLE

Habits (coffee, alcohol, smoking): _____

Sleep (quality, number of hours): _____

Meditation/prayer: _____

OTHER NOTES, IMPRESSIONS, FEELINGS

_____

_____

_____

_____

WEEK 9 / DAY 58   DATE: _____

✛ EXERCISE FOR THE DAY: *weight training*

⬙ WAKE UP: *8-oz glass of water*

▯▤ MORNING SKIN CARE

✗ DIET

BREAKFAST
· Omelet made with 3 egg whites and one yolk
· Sliced tomato
· $^1/_2$ cup blueberries
· Green or black tea or water
· 1 Total Skin & Body Vitamin Packet

LUNCH
· 3 to 6 ounces smoked or grilled salmon
· Green salad with tomatoes, cucumbers, onions and 2 tablespoons
  chickpeas dressed with olive oil, lemon juice, and garlic
· Green or black tea or water
· 1 Total Skin & Body Vitamin Packet

AFTERNOON SNACK
· $^1/_2$ cup low-fat cottage cheese
· 4 small black olives
· 4 endive spears
· Green or black tea or water

DINNER
· 4 to 6 ounces baked or grilled halibut
· 1 cup Chicken-Vegetable Soup*
· Salad of romaine lettuce, chopped avocado, tomato, green onion,
  and celery dressed with olive oil and lemon juice
· Green or black tea or water

BEDTIME SNACK
· 2 ounces sliced roast turkey breast
· 6 whole almonds
· 3 red bell pepper strips
· 2-inch wedge of honeydew melon

* Recipe available in *The Perricone Prescription: A Physician's 28-Day Program for Total Face and Body Rejuvenation.*

EVENING SKIN CARE

RECORD YOUR DAY'S ACTIVITIES, IMPRESSIONS, AND FEELINGS

TAKE A FEW MINUTES TO PRAY, MEDITATE, AND REFLECT

JOURNAL NOTES

THREE THINGS I APPRECIATED IN MY LIFE TODAY:

1. _____

2. _____

3. _____

SKIN

Face and Neck: _____   Fine Lines: _____

Dark Circles: _____   Puffiness: _____

Radiance: _____   Pore Size: _____

Firmness (jawline): _____

BODY

Weight: _____   Tone: _____

Energy: _____   Exercise: _____

MIND

Mood: _____   Stress: _____

Memory: _____   Problem-solving: _____

LIFESTYLE

Habits (coffee, alcohol, smoking): _____

Sleep (quality, number of hours): _____

Meditation/prayer: _____

OTHER NOTES, IMPRESSIONS, FEELINGS

_____

_____

_____

_____

WEEK 9 / DAY 59   DATE: _____

 EXERCISE FOR THE DAY: *aerobics*

WAKE UP: *8-oz glass of water*

MORNING SKIN CARE

DIET

BREAKFAST
· 2 slices turkey bacon
· 6 ounces plain whole milk yogurt
· 1/2 cup strawberries
· Green or black tea or water
· 1 Total Skin & Body Vitamin Packet

LUNCH
· 3- to 4-ounce can water-packed tuna
· 1 cup sliced tomatoes and cucumbers
· 1/2 cup bean salad
· Green or black tea or water
· 1 Total Skin & Body Vitamin Packet

AFTERNOON SNACK
· 2 ounces sliced turkey breast
· 4 hazelnuts
· 1 small pear
· Green or black tea or water

DINNER
· 4 to 6 ounces broiled fillet of salmon. (Make 8 ounces and save
  2 ounces for tomorrow's bedtime snack.)
· 1/4 cup green beans
· Spinach salad with mushrooms, slice of red onion, and 1/4 cup
  chickpeas, dressed with olive oil and lemon juice
· Green or black tea or water

BEDTIME SNACK
· 2 ounces Grilled Chicken Breast*
· 1/4 cup raw cauliflower
· 4 black olives

* Recipe available in *The Perricone Prescription: A Physician's 28-Day Program for
Total Face and Body Rejuvenation.*

EVENING SKIN CARE

RECORD YOUR DAY'S ACTIVITIES, IMPRESSIONS, AND FEELINGS

TAKE A FEW MINUTES TO PRAY, MEDITATE, AND REFLECT

JOURNAL NOTES

THREE THINGS I APPRECIATED IN MY LIFE TODAY:

1. _____
2. _____
3. _____

SKIN

Face and Neck: _____   Fine Lines: _____

Dark Circles: _____   Puffiness: _____

Radiance: _____   Pore Size: _____

Firmness (jawline): _____

BODY

Weight: _____   Tone: _____

Energy: _____   Exercise: _____

MIND

Mood: _____   Stress: _____

Memory: _____   Problem-solving: _____

LIFESTYLE

Habits (coffee, alcohol, smoking): _____

Sleep (quality, number of hours): _____

Meditation/prayer: _____

OTHER NOTES, IMPRESSIONS, FEELINGS

_____

_____

_____

_____

> *Exercise in moderation has a **powerful, positive and anti-inflammatory** effect on our cells.*

WEEK 9 / DAY 60   DATE: _____

 EXERCISE FOR THE DAY: *weight training*

WAKE UP: *8-oz glass of water*

MORNING SKIN CARE

DIET

BREAKFAST
- 1 slice of Canadian bacon or 2 slices turkey bacon
- 2 poached egg whites and one yolk
- ½ cup slow-cooked oatmeal
- ½ cup blueberries
- Green or black tea or water
- 1 Total Skin & Body Vitamin Packet

LUNCH
- 4 ounces grilled chicken salad (with fresh dill, chopped red onion, garlic, and olive oil)
- ½ cup steamed broccoli
- ½ cup strawberries
- Green or black tea or water
- 1 Total Skin & Body Vitamin Packet

AFTERNOON SNACK
- 2 slices roast turkey breast
- 4 cherry tomatoes
- 4 almonds
- Green or black tea or water

DINNER
- 6 ounces broiled fillet of sole, cod, or scrod.
- 8 Oven-Roasted Brussels Sprouts with Apples*
- Romaine lettuce salad with 2 ounces chickpeas, dressed with olive oil, garlic, and lemon juice
- Green or black tea or water

BEDTIME SNACK
- 2 ounces salmon
- 2 tablespoons Cuban Black Bean Salad*

* Recipe available in *The Perricone Prescription: A Physician's 28-Day Program for Total Face and Body Rejuvenation.*

EVENING SKIN CARE

RECORD YOUR DAY'S ACTIVITIES, IMPRESSIONS, AND FEELINGS

TAKE A FEW MINUTES TO PRAY, MEDITATE, AND REFLECT

JOURNAL NOTES

THREE THINGS I APPRECIATED IN MY LIFE TODAY:

1. _____
2. _____
3. _____

SKIN

Face and Neck: _____   Fine Lines: _____

Dark Circles: _____   Puffiness: _____

Radiance: _____   Pore Size: _____

Firmness (jawline): _____

BODY

Weight: _____   Tone: _____

Energy: _____   Exercise: _____

MIND

Mood: _____   Stress: _____

Memory: _____   Problem-solving: _____

LIFESTYLE

Habits (coffee, alcohol, smoking): _____

Sleep (quality, number of hours): _____

Meditation/prayer: _____

OTHER NOTES, IMPRESSIONS, FEELINGS

_____

_____

_____

_____

> *Salmon for breakfast greatly facilitates **weight loss and appetite control.***

Week 9 / Day 61   Date: _____

 Exercise for the day: *aerobics (20 minutes' vigorous walking)*

Wake up: *8-oz glass of water*

Morning skin care

Diet

BREAKFAST
- 4 ounces smoked salmon
- 1/2 cup slow-cooked oatmeal seasoned with cinnamon
- 2 teaspoons chopped almonds
- 2-inch wedge of cantaloupe
- Green or black tea or water
- 1 Total Skin & Body Vitamin Packet

LUNCH
- 4 ounces salmon salad (finely cubed salmon fillet or canned salmon dressed with lemon juice, olive oil, and dill) served on a bed of romaine lettuce
- 1/2 cup lentil soup
- Green or black tea or water
- 1 Total Skin & Body Vitamin Packet

AFTERNOON SNACK
- 2 slices turkey breast
- 1/2 cup strawberries
- 4 hazelnuts
- Green or black tea or water

DINNER
- 1 roast chicken breast (skin removed)
- 1/2 cup grilled zucchini
- 1/2 cup Three Bean Salad*
- Green or black tea or water

BEDTIME SNACK
- 2 ounces drained canned shrimp or tuna
- 3 macadamia nuts
- 3 cherry tomatoes

* Recipe available in *The Perricone Prescription: A Physician's 28-Day Program for Total Face and Body Rejuvenation.*

- **EVENING SKIN CARE**

- **RECORD YOUR DAY'S ACTIVITIES, IMPRESSIONS, AND FEELINGS**

- **TAKE A FEW MINUTES TO PRAY, MEDITATE, AND REFLECT**

JOURNAL NOTES

THREE THINGS I APPRECIATED IN MY LIFE TODAY:

1. _____
2. _____
3. _____

SKIN

Face and Neck: _____ Fine Lines: _____

Dark Circles: _____ Puffiness: _____

Radiance: _____ Pore Size: _____

Firmness (jawline): _____

BODY

Weight: _____ Tone: _____

Energy: _____ Exercise: _____

MIND

Mood: _____ Stress: _____

Memory: _____ Problem-solving: _____

LIFESTYLE

Habits (coffee, alcohol, smoking): _____

Sleep (quality, number of hours): _____

Meditation/prayer: _____

OTHER NOTES, IMPRESSIONS, FEELINGS

_____

_____

_____

_____

WEEK 9 / DAY 62   **DATE:** _____

 EXERCISE FOR THE DAY: *weight training*

WAKE UP: *8-oz glass of water*

MORNING SKIN CARE

DIET

BREAKFAST
· Omelet of 3 egg whites and 1 yolk with a few sliced mushrooms and ¹/₂ cup chopped spinach
· 1 slice Canadian or turkey bacon
· 2-inch wedge of honeydew melon
· Green or black tea or water
· 1 Total Skin & Body Vitamin Packet

LUNCH
· 4 to 6 ounces broiled salmon
· Caesar salad without croutons
· ¹/₂ apple
· Green or black tea or water
· 1 Total Skin & Body Vitamin Packet

AFTERNOON SNACK
· 1 hard-boiled egg
· ¹/₂ cup sliced strawberries
· 3 almonds
· Green or black tea or water

DINNER
· 4 to 6 ounces grilled halibut
· Tossed Greek salad made with romaine lettuce, 3 black olives, 1 ounce feta cheese, ¹/₂ cucumber, 4 cherry tomatoes; dressed with olive oil, lemon juice, and a dash of oregano, mixed to taste
· Steamed or Grilled Asparagus*
· 2-inch wedge of cataloupe
· Green or black tea or water

BEDTIME SNACK
· 2 slices roast turkey or chicken breast
· 4 macadamia nuts
· Small peach or nectarine

* Recipe available in *The Perricone Prescription: A Physician's 28-Day Program for Total Face and Body Rejuvenation.*

EVENING SKIN CARE

RECORD YOUR DAY'S ACTIVITIES, IMPRESSIONS, AND FEELINGS

TAKE A FEW MINUTES TO PRAY, MEDITATE, AND REFLECT

JOURNAL NOTES

THREE THINGS I APPRECIATED IN MY LIFE TODAY:
1. _____
2. _____
3. _____

SKIN

Face and Neck: _____   Fine Lines: _____

Dark Circles: _____   Puffiness: _____

Radiance: _____   Pore Size: _____

Firmness (jawline): _____

BODY

Weight: _____   Tone: _____

Energy: _____   Exercise: _____

MIND

Mood: _____   Stress: _____

Memory: _____   Problem-solving: _____

LIFESTYLE

Habits (coffee, alcohol, smoking): _____

Sleep (quality, number of hours): _____

Meditation/prayer: _____

OTHER NOTES, IMPRESSIONS, FEELINGS

_____

_____

_____

_____

> *A diet rich in **extra virgin olive oil** increases the skin's ability to maintain moisture, lowers blood pressure, prevents osteoporosis, reduces the risk of certain cancers… and much more.*

WEEK 9 / DAY 63   DATE: _____

EXERCISE FOR THE DAY: *relaxation (you've earned it!)*

WAKE UP: *8-oz glass of water*

MORNING SKIN CARE

DIET

BREAKFAST
· 3 to 6 ounces broiled salmon
· $1/2$ cup slow-cooked oatmeal
· 2-inch wedge of cantaloupe
· Green or black tea or water
· 1 Total Skin & Body Vitamin Packet

LUNCH
· Crabmeat salad made with a 6-ounce can of crabmeat, 1 chopped scallion, 1 chopped celery rib; dress with $1/4$ cup yogurt, juice of $1/2$ lemon; serve inside $1/2$ avocado
· 1 cup strawberries
· Green or black tea or water
· 1 Total Skin & Body Vitamin Packet

AFTERNOON SNACK
· $1/2$ cup cottage cheese
· 4 almonds
· 1 apple
· Green or black tea or water

DINNER
· Grilled chicken breast*
· $3/4$ cup roasted or sautéed mushrooms and Sautéed Zucchini or Summer Squash*
· Romaine lettuce salad, sliced tomatoes, fresh basil with 1 ounce grated Parmesan cheese, dressed with olive oil and lemon juice, mixed to taste
· Green or black tea or water

BEDTIME SNACK
· 2 slices of turkey breast
· 3 olives
· 1 pear

* Recipe available in *The Perricone Prescription: A Physician's 28-Day Program for Total Face and Body Rejuvenation.*

Evening skin care

Record your day's activities, impressions, and feelings

Take a few minutes to pray, meditate, and reflect

Journal Notes

THREE THINGS I APPRECIATED IN MY LIFE TODAY:
1. _____
2. _____
3. _____

SKIN

Face and Neck: _____ Fine Lines: _____

Dark Circles: _____ Puffiness: _____

Radiance: _____ Pore Size: _____

Firmness (jawline): _____

BODY

Weight: _____ Tone: _____

Energy: _____ Exercise: _____

MIND

Mood: _____ Stress: _____

Memory: _____ Problem-solving: _____

LIFESTYLE

Habits (coffee, alcohol, smoking): _____

Sleep (quality, number of hours): _____

Meditation/prayer: _____

OTHER NOTES, IMPRESSIONS, FEELINGS

_____

_____

_____

_____

> *Alpha lipoic acid is a **natural substance** found in our bodies—and it is one of the most powerful anti-aging, antioxidant, anti-inflammatories available.*

WEEK 10 / DAY 64   DATE: _____

✚ **EXERCISE FOR THE DAY:** *aerobics (20 minutes' vigorous walking)*

💧 **WAKE UP:** *8-oz glass of water*

🧴 **MORNING SKIN CARE**

✗ **DIET**

BREAKFAST
- 2 slices Canadian bacon, ham, or turkey bacon
- 1/2 cup plain cottage cheese
- 1/2 cup blueberries
- Green or black tea or water
- 1 Total Skin & Body Vitamin Packet

LUNCH
- 3- to 4-ounce can water-packed tuna
- 1/2 cup lentil soup
- Romaine lettuce salad topped with chopped tomato and red onion; dress with olive oil and lemon
- Green or black tea or water
- 1 Total Skin & Body Vitamin Packet

AFTERNOON SNACK
- 2 ounces smoked salmon
- 3 hazelnuts
- 2-inch wedge cantaloupe
- Green or black tea or water

DINNER
- 6 ounces Scallops with Garlic and Parsley* (cook 8 ounces and save 2 ounces for tomorrow's lunch)
- Mediterranean Chopped Salad* with 1/2 cup chickpeas
- 1/2 cup cooked green beans
- Green or black tea or water

BEDTIME SNACK
- 2 slices turkey breast
- 4 green olives
- 1 apple

* Recipe available in *The Perricone Prescription: A Physician's 28-Day Program for Total Face and Body Rejuvenation.*

- ☐▤ EVENING SKIN CARE
- 📖 RECORD YOUR DAY'S ACTIVITIES, IMPRESSIONS, AND FEELINGS
- ☁ TAKE A FEW MINUTES TO PRAY, MEDITATE, AND REFLECT

JOURNAL NOTES

THREE THINGS I APPRECIATED IN MY LIFE TODAY:

1. _____
2. _____
3. _____

SKIN

Face and Neck: _____   Fine Lines: _____

Dark Circles: _____   Puffiness: _____

Radiance: _____   Pore Size: _____

Firmness (jawline): _____

BODY

Weight: _____   Tone: _____

Energy: _____   Exercise: _____

MIND

Mood: _____   Stress: _____

Memory: _____   Problem-solving: _____

LIFESTYLE

Habits (coffee, alcohol, smoking): _____

Sleep (quality, number of hours): _____

Meditation/prayer: _____

OTHER NOTES, IMPRESSIONS, FEELINGS

_____

_____

_____

_____

> *Even the busiest person can find time during the day*
> *for a **twenty-minute walk**.*

WEEK 10 / DAY 65   DATE: _____

 EXERCISE FOR THE DAY: *weight training*

WAKE UP: *8-oz glass of water*

MORNING SKIN CARE

DIET

BREAKFAST
· Egg white omelet made with 3 to 4 egg whites and one yolk (add a few sliced mushrooms, if desired)
· 1/2 cup slow-cooked oatmeal
· 3 hazelnuts
· Green or black tea or water
· 1 Total Skin & Body Vitamin Packet

LUNCH
· Scallop salad (2 ounces scallops from previous night's dinner); dressed with olive oil, lemon juice, chopped red onion, and dill
· 1/2 cup Three Bean Salad*
· Green or black tea or water
· 1 Total Skin & Body Vitamin Packet

AFTERNOON SNACK
· 2 ounces smoked salmon
· 4 black olives
· 3 endive spears
· Green or black tea or water

DINNER
· 6 ounces grilled salmon
· 1/2 cup Cuban Black Bean Soup*
· Romaine salad dressed with olive oil and lemon juice
· 1/2 cup berries
· Green or black tea or water

BEDTIME SNACK
· 6 ounces plain whole milk yogurt or cottage cheese
· 1/2 cup strawberries
· 4 macadamia nuts

* Recipe available in *The Perricone Prescription: A Physician's 28-Day Program for Total Face and Body Rejuvenation.*

Evening skin care

Record your day's activities, impressions, and feelings

Take a few minutes to pray, meditate, and reflect

Journal Notes

THREE THINGS I APPRECIATED IN MY LIFE TODAY:
1. _____
2. _____
3. _____

SKIN

Face and Neck: _____   Fine Lines: _____

Dark Circles: _____   Puffiness: _____

Radiance: _____   Pore Size: _____

Firmness (jawline): _____

BODY

Weight: _____   Tone: _____

Energy: _____   Exercise: _____

MIND

Mood: _____   Stress: _____

Memory: _____   Problem-solving: _____

LIFESTYLE

Habits (coffee, alcohol, smoking): _____

Sleep (quality, number of hours): _____

Meditation/prayer: _____

OTHER NOTES, IMPRESSIONS, FEELINGS

_____

_____

_____

_____

WEEK 10 / DAY 66   DATE: _____

 EXERCISE FOR THE DAY: *aerobics*

WAKE UP: *8-oz glass of water*

MORNING SKIN CARE

DIET

BREAKFAST
- 2 slices turkey bacon
- 1 cup plain whole milk yogurt
- 1/2 cup strawberries
- 3 almonds
- Green or black tea or water
- 1 Total Skin & Body Vitamin Packet

LUNCH
- 4 to 6 ounces grilled chicken
- 1/2 cup vegetable barley soup
- Large green salad with sliced tomatoes
- 2-inch wedge of cantaloupe
- Green or black tea or water
- 1 Total Skin & Body Vitamin Packet

AFTERNOON SNACK
- 1 hard-boiled egg
- 2-inch wedge of cantaloupe
- 4 almonds
- Green or black tea or water

DINNER
- 6 ounces Scallops with Garlic and Parsley*
- Mediterranean Chopped Salad* with 1/2 cup chickpeas
- 1/2 cup cooked green beans
- Green or black tea or water

BEDTIME SNACK
- 2 slices turkey breast
- 4 green olives
- 1 apple

* Recipe available in *The Perricone Prescription: A Physician's 28-Day Program for Total Face and Body Rejuvenation.*

EVENING SKIN CARE

RECORD YOUR DAY'S ACTIVITIES, IMPRESSIONS, AND FEELINGS

TAKE A FEW MINUTES TO PRAY, MEDITATE, AND REFLECT

JOURNAL NOTES

THREE THINGS I APPRECIATED IN MY LIFE TODAY:
1. _____
2. _____
3. _____

SKIN
Face and Neck: _____   Fine Lines: _____

Dark Circles: _____   Puffiness: _____

Radiance: _____   Pore Size: _____

Firmness (jawline): _____

BODY
Weight: _____   Tone: _____

Energy: _____   Exercise: _____

MIND
Mood: _____   Stress: _____

Memory: _____   Problem-solving: _____

LIFESTYLE
Habits (coffee, alcohol, smoking): _____

Sleep (quality, number of hours): _____

Meditation/prayer: _____

OTHER NOTES, IMPRESSIONS, FEELINGS
_____
_____
_____
_____

> *Watch portion size—even good foods can cause an insulin response if we eat too much at one sitting.*

WEEK 10 / DAY 67   DATE: _____

EXERCISE FOR THE DAY: *weight training*

WAKE UP: *8-oz glass of water*

MORNING SKIN CARE

DIET

BREAKFAST
- 4 ounces smoked salmon
- 3 ounces plain whole milk yogurt
- 1 tomato slice
- 1/4 cantaloupe
- Green or black tea or water
- 1 Total Skin & Body Vitamin Packet

LUNCH
- 6 ounces canned crabmeat dressed with 1 tablespoon mayonnaise
- 1/2 cup lentil soup
- Large romaine lettuce salad dressed with olive oil and lemon to taste
- Green or black tea or water
- 1 Total Skin & Body Vitamin Packet

AFTERNOON SNACK
- 1 hard-boiled egg
- 4 cherry tomatoes
- 4 macadamia nuts
- Green or black tea or water

DINNER
- 6 ounces roast chicken breast (cook 8 ounces and save 2 ounces for tomorrow's lunch)
- 1/2 cup Manhattan Clam Chowder*
- 1/2 cup grilled eggplant topped with sliced tomato and 1 tablespoon grated Parmesan cheese
- Green or black tea or water

BEDTIME SNACK
- 1/2 cup cottage cheese
- 1/2 cup blueberries
- 4 hazelnuts

* Recipe available in *The Perricone Prescription: A Physician's 28-Day Program for Total Face and Body Rejuvenation.*

EVENING SKIN CARE

RECORD YOUR DAY'S ACTIVITIES, IMPRESSIONS, AND FEELINGS

TAKE A FEW MINUTES TO PRAY, MEDITATE, AND REFLECT

JOURNAL NOTES

THREE THINGS I APPRECIATED IN MY LIFE TODAY:

1. _____
2. _____
3. _____

SKIN

Face and Neck: _____   Fine Lines: _____

Dark Circles: _____   Puffiness: _____

Radiance: _____   Pore Size: _____

Firmness (jawline): _____

BODY

Weight: _____   Tone: _____

Energy: _____   Exercise: _____

MIND

Mood: _____   Stress: _____

Memory: _____   Problem-solving: _____

LIFESTYLE

Habits (coffee, alcohol, smoking): _____

Sleep (quality, number of hours): _____

Meditation/prayer: _____

OTHER NOTES, IMPRESSIONS, FEELINGS

_____

_____

_____

_____

> *An ongoing lack of protein is always **noticeable** in the face first.*

WEEK 10 / DAY 68   DATE: _____

✛ **EXERCISE FOR THE DAY:** *aerobics (20 minutes' vigorous walking)*

💧 **WAKE UP:** *8-oz glass of water*

🧴 **MORNING SKIN CARE**

✗ **DIET**

BREAKFAST
· Scrambled eggs (3 egg whites and 1 yolk) with a little chopped onion and green bell peppers
· 2 slices turkey bacon
· 2-inch wedge cantaloupe
· Green or black tea or water
· 1 Total Skin & Body Vitamin Packet

LUNCH
· 3 to 5 ounces of chicken salad (made with 2 ounces chicken saved from last night's dinner, mixed with chopped red onion and celery, and dressed with 1 tablespoon olive oil and lemon juice) served on a bed of romaine lettuce
· Sliced tomatoes
· 1 cup Chicken-Vegetable Soup*
· Green or black tea or water
· 1 Total Skin & Body Vitamin Packet

AFTERNOON SNACK
· $1/2$ cup plain whole milk yogurt
· $1/2$ cup blueberries
· 1 teaspoon chopped almonds
· Green or black tea or water

DINNER
· 6 ounces grilled salmon
· Salad of romaine lettuce, avocado, and tomato, dressed with olive oil and lemon juice
· Grilled zucchini and mushroom kebabs
· Green or black tea or water

BEDTIME SNACK
· 2 ounces tuna salad (tuna mixed with onion, celery, pepper, and mustard or a touch or mayonnaise, if desired)
· 4 almonds
· 1 pear

* Recipe available in *The Perricone Prescription: A Physician's 28-Day Program for Total Face and Body Rejuvenation.*

EVENING SKIN CARE

RECORD YOUR DAY'S ACTIVITIES, IMPRESSIONS, AND FEELINGS

TAKE A FEW MINUTES TO PRAY, MEDITATE, AND REFLECT

JOURNAL NOTES

THREE THINGS I APPRECIATED IN MY LIFE TODAY:

1. _____
2. _____
3. _____

SKIN

Face and Neck: _____ Fine Lines: _____

Dark Circles: _____ Puffiness: _____

Radiance: _____ Pore Size: _____

Firmness (jawline): _____

BODY

Weight: _____ Tone: _____

Energy: _____ Exercise: _____

MIND

Mood: _____ Stress: _____

Memory: _____ Problem-solving: _____

LIFESTYLE

Habits (coffee, alcohol, smoking): _____

Sleep (quality, number of hours): _____

Meditation/prayer: _____

OTHER NOTES, IMPRESSIONS, FEELINGS

_____

_____

_____

_____

> *Olive oil is one of **nature's greatest gifts** for preserving your health, beauty, and longevity.*

WEEK 10 / DAY 69   DATE: _____

 EXERCISE FOR THE DAY: *aerobics*

WAKE UP: *8-oz glass of water*

MORNING SKIN CARE

DIET

BREAKFAST
- 2 to 4 ounces smoked salmon
- 1/2 cup plain whole milk yogurt
- 1 tablespoon chopped walnuts
- 1/2 cup blueberries
- Green or black tea or water
- 1 Total Skin & Body Vitamin Packet

LUNCH
- Grilled Chicken Breast*
- Green salad topped with 1/2 cup white or navy beans
- Steamed asparagus
- Green or black tea or water
- 1 Total Skin & Body Vitamin Packet

AFTERNOON SNACK
- 1 hard-boiled egg
- 2-inch wedge cantaloupe
- 4 macadamia nuts
- Green or black tea or water

DINNER
- 6 ounces grilled bluefin or albacore tuna steak
- 1/2 cup grilled zucchini, eggplant, and red or green bell peppers lightly drizzled with olive oil and sprinkled with 1 tablespoon Parmesan cheese
- Tomato salsa (use fresh, if possible)
- Green or black tea or water

BEDTIME SNACK
- 2 slices turkey breast
- 4 green olives
- 4 cherry tomatoes

* Recipe available in *The Perricone Prescription: A Physician's 28-Day Program for Total Face and Body Rejuvenation.*

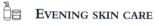 EVENING SKIN CARE

RECORD YOUR DAY'S ACTIVITIES, IMPRESSIONS, AND FEELINGS

TAKE A FEW MINUTES TO PRAY, MEDITATE, AND REFLECT

JOURNAL NOTES

THREE THINGS I APPRECIATED IN MY LIFE TODAY:

1. _____
2. _____
3. _____

SKIN

Face and Neck: _____   Fine Lines: _____

Dark Circles: _____   Puffiness: _____

Radiance: _____   Pore Size: _____

Firmness (jawline): _____

BODY

Weight: _____   Tone: _____

Energy: _____   Exercise: _____

MIND

Mood: _____   Stress: _____

Memory: _____   Problem-solving: _____

LIFESTYLE

Habits (coffee, alcohol, smoking): _____

Sleep (quality, number of hours): _____

Meditation/prayer: _____

OTHER NOTES, IMPRESSIONS, FEELINGS

_____

_____

_____

_____

WEEK 10 / DAY 70   DATE: _____

EXERCISE FOR THE DAY: *relaxation (you've* **REALLY** *earned it!)*

WAKE UP: *8-oz glass of water*

MORNING SKIN CARE

DIET

BREAKFAST
· Omelet made with 3 egg whites, 1 yolk, and a few sliced fresh mushrooms
· $1/2$ cup slow-cooked oatmeal
· 1 teaspoon chopped almonds
· 2-inch wedge cantaloupe
· Green or black tea or water
· 1 Total Skin & Body Vitamin Packet

LUNCH
· 3 to 4 ounces water-packed tuna
· Romaine lettuce salad made with $1/2$ cup white beans, $1/4$ cup crumbled feta cheese, 4 cherry tomatoes, and sliced red onion, dressed with olive oil and lemon juice
· Green or black tea or water
· 1 Total Skin & Body Vitamin Packet

AFTERNOON SNACK
· 1 slice turkey breast
· 4 hazelnuts
· 2-inch wedge cantaloupe
· Green or black tea or water

DINNER
· 4 large shrimp, grilled, broiled, or baked on skewers with mushrooms, onions, and cherry tomatoes
· $1/2$ cup Cuban Black Bean Soup*
· Romaine lettuce salad dressed with olive oil and lemon juice
· Green or black tea or water

BEDTIME SNACK
· 2 slices turkey breast
· 4 green olives
· 4 cherry tomatoes

* Recipe available in *The Perricone Prescription: A Physician's 28-Day Program for Total Face and Body Rejuvenation.*

Eᴠᴇɴɪɴɢ sᴋɪɴ ᴄᴀʀᴇ

Rᴇᴄᴏʀᴅ ʏᴏᴜʀ ᴅᴀʏ's ᴀᴄᴛɪᴠɪᴛɪᴇs, ɪᴍᴘʀᴇssɪᴏɴs, ᴀɴᴅ ꜰᴇᴇʟɪɴɢs

Tᴀᴋᴇ ᴀ ꜰᴇw ᴍɪɴᴜᴛᴇs ᴛᴏ ᴘʀᴀʏ, ᴍᴇᴅɪᴛᴀᴛᴇ, ᴀɴᴅ ʀᴇꜰʟᴇᴄᴛ

Jᴏᴜʀɴᴀʟ Nᴏᴛᴇs

THREE THINGS I APPRECIATED IN MY LIFE TODAY:

1. _____
2. _____
3. _____

SKIN

Face and Neck: _____   Fine Lines: _____

Dark Circles: _____   Puffiness: _____

Radiance: _____   Pore Size: _____

Firmness (jawline): _____

BODY

Weight: _____   Tone: _____

Energy: _____   Exercise: _____

MIND

Mood: _____   Stress: _____

Memory: _____   Problem-solving: _____

LIFESTYLE

Habits (coffee, alcohol, smoking): _____

Sleep (quality, number of hours): _____

Meditation/prayer: _____

OTHER NOTES, IMPRESSIONS, FEELINGS

_____
_____
_____
_____

> *Drinking hard liquor causes inflammatory problems in the body. In short: wine is fine… but **forget the martini**.*

WEEK 11 / DAY 71   DATE: _____

✛ **EXERCISE FOR THE DAY:** *aerobics (20 minutes' vigorous walking)*

💧 **WAKE UP:** *8-oz glass of water*

🧴 **MORNING SKIN CARE**

✗ **DIET**

BREAKFAST
· 2 ounces smoked salmon
· 6 ounces plain whole milk yogurt
· 2-inch wedge cantaloupe
· Green or black tea or water
· 1 Total Skin & Body Vitamin Packet

LUNCH
· 1 6-ounce can shrimp (drained) mixed with 1 tablespoon olive oil and juice of 1/2 lemon, served inside 1/2 avocado
· 1/2 cup cherries
· Green or black tea or water
· 1 Total Skin & Body Vitamin Packet

AFTERNOON SNACK
· 2 ounces sliced turkey or chicken breast
· 4 almonds
· 4 cherry tomatoes
· Green or black tea or water

DINNER
· 4 to 6 ounces baked scrod fillets
· 1/2 cup steamed broccoli or spinach
· Tossed green salad dressed with olive oil and lemon juice
· Green or black tea or water

BEDTIME SNACK
· 1 hard-boiled egg
· 3 celery sticks
· 3 green olives

- **EVENING SKIN CARE**

- **RECORD YOUR DAY'S ACTIVITIES, IMPRESSIONS, AND FEELINGS**

- **TAKE A FEW MINUTES TO PRAY, MEDITATE, AND REFLECT**

JOURNAL NOTES

THREE THINGS I APPRECIATED IN MY LIFE TODAY:

1. _____

2. _____

3. _____

SKIN

Face and Neck: _____   Fine Lines: _____

Dark Circles: _____   Puffiness: _____

Radiance: _____   Pore Size: _____

Firmness (jawline): _____

BODY

Weight: _____   Tone: _____

Energy: _____   Exercise: _____

MIND

Mood: _____   Stress: _____

Memory: _____   Problem-solving: _____

LIFESTYLE

Habits (coffee, alcohol, smoking): _____

Sleep (quality, number of hours): _____

Meditation/prayer: _____

OTHER NOTES, IMPRESSIONS, FEELINGS

_____

_____

_____

_____

> *A **good night's sleep** can help you awake refreshed,*
> *looking radiant and youthful. And, after a good night's sleep,*
> *doesn't the world look better, too?*

WEEK 11 / DAY 72 DATE: _____

EXERCISE FOR THE DAY: *weight training*

WAKE UP: *8-oz glass of water*

MORNING SKIN CARE

 DIET

BREAKFAST
· Omelet made with 2 eggs, fresh herbs, and a few sliced fresh mushrooms
· $^1/_2$ cup slow-cooked oatmeal
· 3 hazelnuts
· $^1/_2$ cup blueberries
· Green or black tea or water
· 1 Total Skin & Body Vitamin Packet

LUNCH
· 3 to 6 ounces canned salmon mixed with 1 teaspoon mayonnaise
· Green salad with sliced tomatoes, cucumbers, and 2 tablespoons chickpeas; dressed with olive oil and lemon juice
· 2-inch wedge honeydew melon
· Green or black tea or water
· 1 Total Skin & Body Vitamin Packet

AFTERNOON SNACK
· 6 ounces plain whole milk yogurt
· 3 hazelnuts
· $^1/_4$ cup fresh berries
· Green or black tea or water

DINNER
· 4 to 6 ounces baked or grilled trout
· Three-bean salad made with $^1/_2$ cup lentils, $^1/_2$ cup green beans, and $^1/_2$ cup chickpeas; dressed with olive oil and lemon juice
· $^1/_2$ cup steamed and mashed turnip
· 1 pear
· Green or black tea or water

BEDTIME SNACK
· 2 ounces sliced roast turkey breast
· 4 almonds
· 3 radishes

EVENING SKIN CARE

RECORD YOUR DAY'S ACTIVITIES, IMPRESSIONS, AND FEELINGS

TAKE A FEW MINUTES TO PRAY, MEDITATE, AND REFLECT

JOURNAL NOTES

THREE THINGS I APPRECIATED IN MY LIFE TODAY:

1. _____
2. _____
3. _____

SKIN

Face and Neck: _____   Fine Lines: _____

Dark Circles: _____   Puffiness: _____

Radiance: _____   Pore Size: _____

Firmness (jawline): _____

BODY

Weight: _____   Tone: _____

Energy: _____   Exercise: _____

MIND

Mood: _____   Stress: _____

Memory: _____   Problem-solving: _____

LIFESTYLE

Habits (coffee, alcohol, smoking): _____

Sleep (quality, number of hours): _____

Meditation/prayer: _____

OTHER NOTES, IMPRESSIONS, FEELINGS

_____

_____

_____

_____

WEEK 11 / DAY 73　　　DATE: _____

 EXERCISE FOR THE DAY: *aerobics*

WAKE UP: *8-oz glass of water*

MORNING SKIN CARE

DIET

BREAKFAST
- 2 slices turkey bacon
- $\frac{1}{2}$ cup slow-cooked oatmeal
- 3 hazelnuts
- $\frac{1}{2}$ grapefruit
- Green or black tea or water
- 1 Total Skin & Body Vitamin Packet

LUNCH
- 3- to 4-ounce can tuna or sardines
- 1 cup sliced tomatoes and cucumbers
- $\frac{1}{2}$ cup lentil soup
- Green or black tea or water
- 1 Total Skin & Body Vitamin Packet

AFTERNOON SNACK
- 6 ounces plain whole milk yogurt
- 4 chopped almonds
- 1 small apple
- Green or black tea or water

DINNER
- 4 to 6 ounces broiled fillet of salmon
- 1 cup steamed asparagus
- Romaine lettuce salad with $\frac{1}{4}$ cup chickpeas; dressed with olive oil and lemon juice
- Green or black tea or water

BEDTIME SNACK
- 2 ounces sliced turkey or chicken breast
- 4 black olives
- 1 kiwi fruit

EVENING SKIN CARE

RECORD YOUR DAY'S ACTIVITIES, IMPRESSIONS, AND FEELINGS

TAKE A FEW MINUTES TO PRAY, MEDITATE, AND REFLECT

JOURNAL NOTES

THREE THINGS I APPRECIATED IN MY LIFE TODAY:

1. _____
2. _____
3. _____

SKIN

Face and Neck: _____   Fine Lines: _____

Dark Circles: _____   Puffiness: _____

Radiance: _____   Pore Size: _____

Firmness (jawline): _____

BODY

Weight: _____   Tone: _____

Energy: _____   Exercise: _____

MIND

Mood: _____   Stress: _____

Memory: _____   Problem-solving: _____

LIFESTYLE

Habits (coffee, alcohol, smoking): _____

Sleep (quality, number of hours): _____

Meditation/prayer: _____

OTHER NOTES, IMPRESSIONS, FEELINGS

_____

_____

_____

_____

> ***Brain function*** *is intimately tied to our essential*
> *fatty acid intake.*

Week 11 / Day 74   Date: _____

 Exercise for the day: *aerobics (20 minutes' vigorous walking)*

Wake up: *8-oz glass of water*

Morning skin care

Diet

BREAKFAST
· 2 links turkey sausage
· 1 soft-boiled egg
· 1/2 cup slow-cooked oatmeal
· 2-inch wedge cantaloupe
· Green or black tea or water
· 1 Total Skin & Body Vitamin Packet

LUNCH
· 4 ounces chicken salad (diced chicken breast mixed with fresh dill,
  chopped red onion, chopped celery; dressed with olive oil and lemon
  juice) served on a bed of romaine lettuce
· 4 hazelnuts
· 1 apple
· Green or black tea or water
· 1 Total Skin & Body Vitamin Packet

AFTERNOON SNACK
· 6 ounces plain whole milk yogurt
· 4 almonds
· 1/4 cup fresh cherries
· Green or black tea or water

DINNER
· 6 ounces broiled fillet of sole, cod, or scrod. (Make 8 ounces and save
  2 ounces for tomorrow's bedtime snack.)
· 1 cup steamed spinach
· Romaine lettuce salad with 1/4 cup chickpeas; dressed with olive oil,
  minced garlic, and lemon juice
· 1/2 cup mixed fresh berries
· Green or black tea or water

BEDTIME SNACK
· 3-ounce can tuna
· 4 macadamia nuts
· 1 pear

EVENING SKIN CARE

RECORD YOUR DAY'S ACTIVITIES, IMPRESSIONS, AND FEELINGS

TAKE A FEW MINUTES TO PRAY, MEDITATE, AND REFLECT

JOURNAL NOTES

THREE THINGS I APPRECIATED IN MY LIFE TODAY:
1. _____
2. _____
3. _____

SKIN

Face and Neck: _____ Fine Lines: _____

Dark Circles: _____ Puffiness: _____

Radiance: _____ Pore Size: _____

Firmness (jawline): _____

BODY

Weight: _____ Tone: _____

Energy: _____ Exercise: _____

MIND

Mood: _____ Stress: _____

Memory: _____ Problem-solving: _____

LIFESTYLE

Habits (coffee, alcohol, smoking): _____

Sleep (quality, number of hours): _____

Meditation/prayer: _____

OTHER NOTES, IMPRESSIONS, FEELINGS

_____

_____

_____

_____

WEEK 11 / DAY 75   DATE: _____

✛ **EXERCISE FOR THE DAY:** *aerobics (20 minutes' vigorous walking)*

💧 **WAKE UP:** *8-oz glass of water*

🧴 **MORNING SKIN CARE**

✗ **DIET**

BREAKFAST
· 3 strips turkey bacon
· ¹/₂ cup slow-cooked oatmeal
· 4 hazelnuts
· 2-inch wedge cantaloupe
· Green or black tea or water
· 1 Total Skin & Body Vitamin Packet

LUNCH
· 4 ounces salmon salad (finely cubed salmon fillet or canned salmon dressed with lemon juice, olive oil, and fresh dill) served on a bed of romaine lettuce
· ¹/₂ cup lentil soup
· 1 kiwi fruit
· Green or black tea or water
· 1 Total Skin & Body Vitamin Packet

AFTERNOON SNACK
· 2 slices turkey breast
· ¹/₄ cup fresh strawberries
· 4 hazelnuts
· Green or black tea or water

DINNER
· 6 ounces baked chicken breast (skin removed)
· ¹/₂ cup sautéed zucchini or summer squash topped with 4 chopped almonds
· ¹/₂ cup Three Bean Salad*
· 2-inch wedge honeydew melon
· Green or black tea or water

BEDTIME SNACK
· 2 ounces cold fillet of sole, cod, or scrod
· 3 macadamia nuts
· 3 cherry tomatoes

* Recipe available in *The Perricone Prescription: A Physician's 28-Day Program for Total Face and Body Rejuvenation.*

☐ **Evening skin care**

☐ **Record your day's activities, impressions, and feelings**

☐ **Take a few minutes to pray, meditate, and reflect**

Journal Notes

THREE THINGS I APPRECIATED IN MY LIFE TODAY:
1. _____
2. _____
3. _____

SKIN

Face and Neck: _____   Fine Lines: _____

Dark Circles: _____   Puffiness: _____

Radiance: _____   Pore Size: _____

Firmness (jawline): _____

BODY

Weight: _____   Tone: _____

Energy: _____   Exercise: _____

MIND

Mood: _____   Stress: _____

Memory: _____   Problem-solving: _____

LIFESTYLE

Habits (coffee, alcohol, smoking): _____

Sleep (quality, number of hours): _____

Meditation/prayer: _____

OTHER NOTES, IMPRESSIONS, FEELINGS

_____

_____

_____

_____

> *Exercise is vital for your health. Studies have shown that* **exercise benefits the skin** *in much the same way it improves bone and muscle quality.*

WEEK 11 / DAY 76   DATE: _____

 EXERCISE FOR THE DAY: *weight training*

WAKE UP: *8-oz glass of water*

MORNING SKIN CARE

DIET

BREAKFAST
· Omelet made with 2 eggs, 1 ounce crumbled feta cheese, and 1/2 teaspoon fresh dill
· 2 ounces smoked salmon
· 1/2 cup blueberries
· Green or black tea or water
· 1 Total Skin & Body Vitamin Packet

LUNCH
· 4 to 6 ounces broiled turkey burger (no bun)
· 1 cup salad made with cherry tomatoes, sliced cucumbers, and chopped red onion; dressed with olive oil and lemon juice
· 1 apple
· Green or black tea or water
· 1 Total Skin & Body Vitamin Packet

AFTERNOON SNACK
· 6 ounces plain whole milk yogurt
· 1/4 cup sliced fresh strawberries
· Green or black tea or water

DINNER
· 4 to 6 ounces baked or grilled halibut or sea bass
· 1 cup steamed asparagus
· Romaine lettuce salad with 1/4 cup chickpeas, dressed with olive oil and lemon juice
· 2-inch wedge cantaloupe
· Green or black tea or water

BEDTIME SNACK
· 2 slices roast turkey or chicken breast
· 4 macadamia nuts
· 1/4 cup fresh cherries

* Recipe available in *The Perricone Prescription: A Physician's 28-Day Program for Total Face and Body Rejuvenation.*

EVENING SKIN CARE

RECORD YOUR DAY'S ACTIVITIES, IMPRESSIONS, AND FEELINGS

TAKE A FEW MINUTES TO PRAY, MEDITATE, AND REFLECT

JOURNAL NOTES

THREE THINGS I APPRECIATED IN MY LIFE TODAY:
1. _____
2. _____
3. _____

SKIN

Face and Neck: _____   Fine Lines: _____

Dark Circles: _____   Puffiness: _____

Radiance: _____   Pore Size: _____

Firmness (jawline): _____

BODY

Weight: _____   Tone: _____

Energy: _____   Exercise: _____

MIND

Mood: _____   Stress: _____

Memory: _____   Problem-solving: _____

LIFESTYLE

Habits (coffee, alcohol, smoking): _____

Sleep (quality, number of hours): _____

Meditation/prayer: _____

OTHER NOTES, IMPRESSIONS, FEELINGS

_____

_____

_____

_____

> *All skin tones are vulnerable to damage from the sun's ultraviolet rays.* **Applying sunscreen** *at the start of your day should be as automatic as combing your hair.*

WEEK 11 / DAY 77   DATE: _____

EXERCISE FOR THE DAY: *relaxation*

 WAKE UP: *8-oz glass of water*

MORNING SKIN CARE

DIET

BREAKFAST
- 3 ounces broiled salmon
- ¹/₂ cup slow-cooked oatmeal
- 2-inch wedge cantaloupe
- Green or black tea or water
- 1 Total Skin & Body Vitamin Packet

LUNCH
- 6-ounce can of tuna or sardines
- Greek salad with romaine lettuce, 3 black olives, 1 ounce feta cheese, ¹/₂ sliced cucumber, 4 cherry tomatoes; dress with olive oil, lemon juice, dash of oregano; toss
- ¹/₂ cup mixed fresh berries
- Green or black tea or water
- 1 Total Skin & Body Vitamin Packet

AFTERNOON SNACK
- ¹/₂ cup plain cottage cheese
- 4 hazelnuts
- 1 apple
- Green or black tea or water

DINNER
- Chicken Stir Fry (6 ounces chicken breast chopped into 1-inch strips; ¹/₄ cup each sliced mushrooms, chopped onions, water chestnuts, chopped almonds, bamboo shoots, bok choy or celery, and mung bean sprouts; toss together and stir fry in olive oil)
- Romaine lettuce salad dressed with olive oil and lemon juice
- 2-inch wedge cantaloupe
- Green or black tea or water

BEDTIME SNACK
- 2 slices turkey breast
- 3 olives
- 1 pear

EVENING SKIN CARE

RECORD YOUR DAY'S ACTIVITIES, IMPRESSIONS, AND FEELINGS

TAKE A FEW MINUTES TO PRAY, MEDITATE, AND REFLECT

JOURNAL NOTES

THREE THINGS I APPRECIATED IN MY LIFE TODAY:

1. _____

2. _____

3. _____

SKIN

Face and Neck: _____   Fine Lines: _____

Dark Circles: _____   Puffiness: _____

Radiance: _____   Pore Size: _____

Firmness (jawline): _____

BODY

Weight: _____   Tone: _____

Energy: _____   Exercise: _____

MIND

Mood: _____   Stress: _____

Memory: _____   Problem-solving: _____

LIFESTYLE

Habits (coffee, alcohol, smoking): _____

Sleep (quality, number of hours): _____

Meditation/prayer: _____

OTHER NOTES, IMPRESSIONS, FEELINGS

_____

_____

_____

_____

> *Food is much more than just a life-giving and life-sustaining substance—it is our **single most powerful** anti-aging tool.*

WEEK 12 / DAY 78   DATE: _____

 EXERCISE FOR THE DAY: *aerobics (20 minutes' vigorous walking)*

WAKE UP: *8-oz glass of water*

MORNING SKIN CARE

DIET

BREAKFAST
- 2 links turkey sausage
- 1 soft-boiled egg
- 1/2 grapefruit
- Green or black tea or water
- 1 Total Skin & Body Vitamin Packet

LUNCH
- 6-ounce canned crabmeat mixed with 1 teaspoon mayonnaise and 1 chopped celery stalk
- 1/2 cup lentil soup
- 1 apple
- Green or black tea or water
- 1 Total Skin & Body Vitamin Packet

AFTERNOON SNACK
- 2 ounces smoked salmon
- 2-inch wedge cantaloupe
- Green or black tea or water

DINNER
- 6 ounces scallops sautéed with minced garlic in olive oil. (Cook 8 ounces and save 2 ounces for tomorrow's lunch.)
- 1/2 cup steamed broccoli
- 1/4 cup fresh cherries
- Green or black tea or water

BEDTIME SNACK
- 6 ounces plain whole milk yogurt
- 4 hazelnuts
- 1/4 cup blueberries

EVENING SKIN CARE

RECORD YOUR DAY'S ACTIVITIES, IMPRESSIONS, AND FEELINGS

TAKE A FEW MINUTES TO PRAY, MEDITATE, AND REFLECT

JOURNAL NOTES

THREE THINGS I APPRECIATED IN MY LIFE TODAY:

1. _____
2. _____
3. _____

SKIN

Face and Neck: _____ Fine Lines: _____

Dark Circles: _____ Puffiness: _____

Radiance: _____ Pore Size: _____

Firmness (jawline): _____

BODY

Weight: _____ Tone: _____

Energy: _____ Exercise: _____

MIND

Mood: _____ Stress: _____

Memory: _____ Problem-solving: _____

LIFESTYLE

Habits (coffee, alcohol, smoking): _____

Sleep (quality, number of hours): _____

Meditation/prayer: _____

OTHER NOTES, IMPRESSIONS, FEELINGS

_____

_____

_____

_____

> *The **fountain of youth** did not spew forth diet soda or orange juice—it's always been good old H_2O.*

WEEK 12 / DAY 79 — DATE: _____

EXERCISE FOR THE DAY: *weight training*

WAKE UP: *8-oz glass of water*

MORNING SKIN CARE

DIET

BREAKFAST
· Vegetable omelet made with 2 eggs and $1/4$ cup each chopped onions, sliced mushrooms, and chopped green pepper
· $1/2$ cup slow-cooked oatmeal
· 3 hazelnuts
· $1/2$ grapefruit
· Green or black tea or water
· 1 Total Skin & Body Vitamin Packet

LUNCH
· Scallop salad made with 2 ounces scallops (from previous night's dinner), chopped red onion, 3 chopped black olives and fresh dill, dressed with olive oil and lemon juice
· 2-inch wedge honeydew melon
· Green or black tea or water
· 1 Total Skin & Body Vitamin Packet

AFTERNOON SNACK
· 6 ounces plain whole milk yogurt
· $1/4$ cup fresh blueberries, blackberries, or raspberries
· 3 macadamia nuts
· Green or black tea or water

DINNER
· 6 ounces grilled salmon
· $1/2$ cup lentil soup
· Romaine lettuce salad dressed with olive oil and lemon juice
· $1/2$ cup fresh cherries
· Green or black tea or water

BEDTIME SNACK
· $1/2$ cup plain cottage cheese
· 3 strawberries
· 4 hazelnuts

EVENING SKIN CARE

RECORD YOUR DAY'S ACTIVITIES, IMPRESSIONS, AND FEELINGS

TAKE A FEW MINUTES TO PRAY, MEDITATE, AND REFLECT

JOURNAL NOTES

THREE THINGS I APPRECIATED IN MY LIFE TODAY:

1. _____

2. _____

3. _____

SKIN

Face and Neck: _____   Fine Lines: _____

Dark Circles: _____   Puffiness: _____

Radiance: _____   Pore Size: _____

Firmness (jawline): _____

BODY

Weight: _____   Tone: _____

Energy: _____   Exercise: _____

MIND

Mood: _____   Stress: _____

Memory: _____   Problem-solving: _____

LIFESTYLE

Habits (coffee, alcohol, smoking): _____

Sleep (quality, number of hours): _____

Meditation/prayer: _____

OTHER NOTES, IMPRESSIONS, FEELINGS

_____

_____

_____

_____

WEEK 12 / DAY 80   DATE: _____

 EXERCISE FOR THE DAY: *aerobics (20 minutes' vigorous walking)*

WAKE UP: *8-oz glass of water*

MORNING SKIN CARE

DIET

BREAKFAST
- 2 links turkey sausage
- 1 poached egg
- 3 almonds
- 2-inch wedge cantaloupe
- Green or black tea or water
- 1 Total Skin & Body Vitamin Packet

LUNCH
- 4 to 6 ounces grilled chicken breast
- Romaine lettuce salad with sliced tomatoes and $1/4$ cup chickpeas; dressed with olive oil and lemon juice
- $1/2$ cup fresh cherries
- Green or black tea or water
- 1 Total Skin & Body Vitamin Packet

AFTERNOON SNACK
- 6 ounces plain whole milk yogurt
- 4 hazelnuts
- 1 kiwi fruit
- Green or black tea or water

DINNER
- 6 ounces broiled trout
- Mixed three-leaf salad (arugula, radicchio, and endive) dressed with olive oil and lemon juice
- $1/2$ cup green beans garnished with chopped almonds
- Green or black tea or water

BEDTIME SNACK
- 2 slices chicken or turkey breast
- 4 macadamia nuts
- 1 small pear

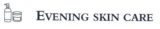

EVENING SKIN CARE

RECORD YOUR DAY'S ACTIVITIES, IMPRESSIONS, AND FEELINGS

TAKE A FEW MINUTES TO PRAY, MEDITATE, AND REFLECT

JOURNAL NOTES

THREE THINGS I APPRECIATED IN MY LIFE TODAY:
1. _____
2. _____
3. _____

SKIN

Face and Neck: _____   Fine Lines: _____

Dark Circles: _____   Puffiness: _____

Radiance: _____   Pore Size: _____

Firmness (jawline): _____

BODY

Weight: _____   Tone: _____

Energy: _____   Exercise: _____

MIND

Mood: _____   Stress: _____

Memory: _____   Problem-solving: _____

LIFESTYLE

Habits (coffee, alcohol, smoking): _____

Sleep (quality, number of hours): _____

Meditation/prayer: _____

OTHER NOTES, IMPRESSIONS, FEELINGS

_____
_____
_____
_____

> *A diet rich in **high quality protein** will firm up the face and body in a matter of weeks.*

WEEK 12 / DAY 81   DATE: _____

 EXERCISE FOR THE DAY: *weight training*

WAKE UP: *8-oz glass of water*

MORNING SKIN CARE

DIET

BREAKFAST
· 4 ounces smoked salmon
· 1 slice tomato
· ½ grapefruit
· Green or black tea or water
· 1 Total Skin & Body Vitamin Packet

LUNCH
· Crabmeat salad (1 6-ounce can of crabmeat mixed with 1 chopped scallion, 1 chopped celery rib, ¼ cup plain yogurt and juice of ½ lemon) served inside ½ avocado
· ½ cup lentil soup
· Green or black tea or water
· 1 Total Skin & Body Vitamin Packet

AFTERNOON SNACK
· 1 hard-boiled egg
· 4 cherry tomatoes
· 4 macadamia nuts
· Green or black tea or water

DINNER
· 6 ounces baked turkey breast.
· 1 small eggplant, sliced and grilled, topped with sliced tomato and 1 tablespoon grated Parmesan cheese
· 1 apple
· Green or black tea or water

BEDTIME SNACK
· 6 ounces plain whole milk yogurt
· 4 hazelnuts
· ¼ cup blueberries

EVENING SKIN CARE

RECORD YOUR DAY'S ACTIVITIES, IMPRESSIONS, AND FEELINGS

TAKE A FEW MINUTES TO PRAY, MEDITATE, AND REFLECT

JOURNAL NOTES

THREE THINGS I APPRECIATED IN MY LIFE TODAY:

1. _____
2. _____
3. _____

SKIN

Face and Neck: _____   Fine Lines: _____

Dark Circles: _____   Puffiness: _____

Radiance: _____   Pore Size: _____

Firmness (jawline): _____

BODY

Weight: _____   Tone: _____

Energy: _____   Exercise: _____

MIND

Mood: _____   Stress: _____

Memory: _____   Problem-solving: _____

LIFESTYLE

Habits (coffee, alcohol, smoking): _____

Sleep (quality, number of hours): _____

Meditation/prayer: _____

OTHER NOTES, IMPRESSIONS, FEELINGS

_____

_____

_____

_____

WEEK 12 / DAY 82   DATE: _____

H **EXERCISE FOR THE DAY:** *aerobics (20 minutes' vigorous walking)*

WAKE UP: *8-oz glass of water*

MORNING SKIN CARE

X **DIET**

BREAKFAST
- 2 slices turkey bacon
- 2 soft-boiled eggs
- 2-inch wedge cantaloupe
- Green or black tea or water
- 1 Total Skin & Body Vitamin Packet

LUNCH
- 3 to 5 ounces chicken salad (mix 2 ounces chicken saved from last night's dinner with 1 teaspoon each chopped red onion and celery, 4 chopped hazelnuts, and 1 tablespoon olive oil and lemon juice) served on a bed of romaine lettuce
- 1 pear
- Green or black tea or water
- 1 Total Skin & Body Vitamin Packet

AFTERNOON SNACK
- 6 ounces plain whole milk yogurt
- $1/4$ cup fresh cherries
- 4 hazelnuts
- Green or black tea or water

DINNER
- 6 ounces grilled salmon
- Salad of romaine lettuce, avocado, and tomato, dressed with olive oil and lemon juice
- 1 cup steamed asparagus
- Green or black tea or water

BEDTIME SNACK
- 2 ounces tuna
- 4 green or black olives
- $1/4$ cup blueberries

EVENING SKIN CARE

RECORD YOUR DAY'S ACTIVITIES, IMPRESSIONS, AND FEELINGS

TAKE A FEW MINUTES TO PRAY, MEDITATE, AND REFLECT

JOURNAL NOTES

THREE THINGS I APPRECIATED IN MY LIFE TODAY:

1. _____
2. _____
3. _____

SKIN

Face and Neck: _____   Fine Lines: _____

Dark Circles: _____   Puffiness: _____

Radiance: _____   Pore Size: _____

Firmness (jawline): _____

BODY

Weight: _____   Tone: _____

Energy: _____   Exercise: _____

MIND

Mood: _____   Stress: _____

Memory: _____   Problem-solving: _____

LIFESTYLE

Habits (coffee, alcohol, smoking): _____

Sleep (quality, number of hours): _____

Meditation/prayer: _____

OTHER NOTES, IMPRESSIONS, FEELINGS

_____

_____

_____

_____

> *Researchers in Boston found patients with manic-depressive disorder who had not responded to conventional treatment **improved dramatically** when given a daily four-ounce serving of salmon.*

WEEK 12 / DAY 83   DATE: _____

EXERCISE FOR THE DAY: *aerobics*

WAKE UP: *8-oz glass of water*

MORNING SKIN CARE

DIET

BREAKFAST
- 2 to 4 ounces smoked salmon
- 6 ounces plain whole milk yogurt
- 4 chopped walnuts
- $^1/_2$ grapefruit
- Green or black tea or water
- 1 Total Skin & Body Vitamin Packet

LUNCH
- 6 ounces grilled turkey burger topped with romaine lettuce, sliced tomato, alfalfa sprouts, and red onion (no bun)
- $^1/_2$ cup lentil soup
- 2-inch wedge honeydew melon
- Green or black tea or water
- 1 Total Skin & Body Vitamin Packet

AFTERNOON SNACK
- 2 ounces sliced chicken breast
- 2-inch wedge cantaloupe
- 4 macadamia nuts
- Green or black tea or water

DINNER
- 6 ounces grilled bluefin or albacore tuna steak
- 1 cup steamed spinach
- Romaine lettuce salad tossed with olive oil and lemon juice
- $^1/_4$ cup mixed fresh berries
- Green or black tea or water

BEDTIME SNACK
- 2 slices turkey breast
- 4 green olives
- 4 cherry tomatoes

◫ **EVENING SKIN CARE**

📖 **RECORD YOUR DAY'S ACTIVITIES, IMPRESSIONS, AND FEELINGS**

☁ **TAKE A FEW MINUTES TO PRAY, MEDITATE, AND REFLECT**

JOURNAL NOTES

THREE THINGS I APPRECIATED IN MY LIFE TODAY:

1. _____
2. _____
3. _____

SKIN

Face and Neck: _____   Fine Lines: _____

Dark Circles: _____   Puffiness: _____

Radiance: _____   Pore Size: _____

Firmness (jawline): _____

BODY

Weight: _____   Tone: _____

Energy: _____   Exercise: _____

MIND

Mood: _____   Stress: _____

Memory: _____   Problem-solving: _____

LIFESTYLE

Habits (coffee, alcohol, smoking): _____

Sleep (quality, number of hours): _____

Meditation/prayer: _____

OTHER NOTES, IMPRESSIONS, FEELINGS

_____

_____

_____

_____

> *Once you accept that your **everyday lifestyle choices**
> affect the way you age, you are on your way toward
> restoring youthful looks and vigor.*

WEEK 12 / DAY 84   DATE: _____

 EXERCISE FOR THE DAY: *relaxation*

WAKE UP: *8-oz glass of water*

MORNING SKIN CARE

DIET

BREAKFAST
· 2 ounces smoked salmon
· $^{1}/_{2}$ cup slow-cooked oatmeal
· 2-inch wedge cantaloupe
· Green or black tea or water
· 1 Total Skin & Body Vitamin Packet

LUNCH
· 3 to 4 ounces tuna tossed with $^{1}/_{2}$ cup white beans, 4 cherry tomatoes, and sliced red onion; dress with olive oil and lemon juice and serve on a bed of romaine lettuce
· 1 apple
· Green or black tea or water
· 1 Total Skin & Body Vitamin Packet

AFTERNOON SNACK
· 6 ounces plain whole milk yogurt
· 4 hazelnuts
· $^{1}/_{2}$ grapefruit
· Green or black tea or water

DINNER
· 4 large shrimp, brushed with olive oil and baked
· Salad of romaine lettuce, $^{1}/_{4}$ cup chickpeas, chopped celery, sliced tomato, and sliced avocado; dress with oil and lemon juice
· $^{1}/_{4}$ cup mixed fresh berries
· Green or black tea or water

BEDTIME SNACK
· $^{1}/_{2}$ cup cottage cheese
· 4 hazelnuts
· 1 pear

EVENING SKIN CARE

RECORD YOUR DAY'S ACTIVITIES, IMPRESSIONS, AND FEELINGS

TAKE A FEW MINUTES TO PRAY, MEDITATE, AND REFLECT

JOURNAL NOTES

THREE THINGS I APPRECIATED IN MY LIFE TODAY:

1. _____
2. _____
3. _____

SKIN

Face and Neck: _____   Fine Lines: _____

Dark Circles: _____   Puffiness: _____

Radiance: _____   Pore Size: _____

Firmness (jawline): _____

BODY

Weight: _____   Tone: _____

Energy: _____   Exercise: _____

MIND

Mood: _____   Stress: _____

Memory: _____   Problem-solving: _____

LIFESTYLE

Habits (coffee, alcohol, smoking): _____

Sleep (quality, number of hours): _____

Meditation/prayer: _____

OTHER NOTES, IMPRESSIONS, FEELINGS

_____

_____

_____

_____

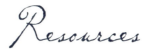

Resources

TOPICAL SKIN CARE PRODUCTS

The following products listed below are available at **www.clinicalcreations.com** or may be ordered by telephone at 888-823-7837. They are also available at

- Sephora
- Nordstrom
- Saks Fifth Avenue
- Neiman Marcus
- Henri Bendel
- Clyde's on Madison

Recommended Topicals—Face

- N.V. PERRICONE M.D. COSMECEUTICALS Alpha Lipoic Acid Nutritive Cleanser
- N.V. PERRICONE M.D. COSMECEUTICALS Alpha Lipoic Acid Face Firming Activator
- N.V. PERRICONE M.D. COSMECEUTICALS Alpha Lipoic Acid Firming Facial Toner
- N.V. PERRICONE M.D. COSMECEUTICALS Vitamin C Ester Concentrated Restorative Cream
- N.V. PERRICONE M.D. COSMECEUTICALS Alpha Lipoic Acid Face Finishing Moisturizer
- N.V. PERRICONE M.D. COSMECEUTICALS Alpha Lipoic Acid Lip Plumper

Recommended Topicals—Eye Area

- N.V. PERRICONE M.D. COSMECEUTICALS Alpha Lipoic Acid Eye Area Therapy

- N.V. PERRICONE M.D. COSMECEUTICALS Vitamin C Ester Eye Area Therapy

Recommended Topicals—Body
- N.V. PERRICONE M.D. COSMECEUTICALS Alpha Lipoic Acid Body Toning Lotion

VITAMIN AND NUTRITIONAL SUPPLEMENTS
Multivitamin packets containing entire Perricone Prescription Program
- N.V. PERRICONE M.D. NUTRICEUTICALS Skin and Total Body Nutritional Supplements (888-823-7837 or **www.clinicalcreations.com**)
- N.V. PERRICONE M.D. NUTRICEUTICALS Weight Management contains the eight fat metabolizers recommended in *The Perricone Prescription*

Other recommended supplements sources
- OPTIMUM HEALTH INTERNATIONAL, 257 East Center Street, Manchester, CT 06040 (1-800-228-1507 or www.optimumhealthintl.com)
- BRONSON PHARMECEUTICALS (phone 800-235-3200 or fax 801-756-5739)
- LIFE EXTENSION, 1100 W. Commercial Blvd., Ft. Lauderdale, FL (1-800-544-4440)

WILD ALASKAN SALMON
Unlike salmon from other parts of the world, no salmon stocks of Alaskan origin are listed as threatened or endangered. Alaskan salmon has been certified by the Marine Stewardship Council as a sustainable resource, one that is carefully managed by the state of Alaska. Alaskan salmon are harvested by families whose livelihood is fishing the cold, clear waters of the North Pacific. For recipes and other information, visit www.alaskaseafood.org or call the Alaska Seafood Marketing Institute (800-806-2497).

Prepackaged and ready-to-ship Alaskan Salmon

An Alaskan company, Vital Choice, has put together a package for anyone wanting to follow the Perricone Prescription.

Dr. Perricone's 28-day diet package from Vital Choice contains the following products:
- Sixteen 6-ounce skinless, boneless sockeye salmon portions
- Six 6-ounce smoked sockeye salmon portions
- Four 6-ounce skinless, boneless halibut portions
- Two 4-ounce Nova Scotia style sliced sockeye lox
- Six 3.75-ounce cans wild red sockeye salmon (easy-open)
- Bonus item: Ten ½-cup portions wild organic blueberries

Vital Choice salmon is
- Natural and pure
- Rich in antioxidants and long chain omega-3s
- Harvested only from sustainable fisheries
- Individually vacuum sealed in convenient 6-ounce skinless, boneless portions
- Carefully packaged and shipped to your home in a sturdy, reusable insulated container

$195.00 for initial order; $185.00 for second and subsequent orders shipped to the same address. 14-day "Sampler Pack" available for $120.00. Shipping and handling included on all orders over $100. Call 800-60-VITAL (800-608-4825) or visit www.vitalchoice.com.

MEDITATIVE/INSPIRATIONAL BOOKS
- *A New You: Words to Soothe the Body, Mind, and Spirit*, by Catherine Galasso-Vigorito (Adams Media Corporation)
- *The Healing Power of Pets: Harnessing the Ability of Pets to Make and Keep People Happy and Healthy*, by Marty Becker, DVM (Hyperion)
- *The Four Agreements: A Practical Guide to Personal Freedom*, by Don Miguel Ruiz (Amer-Allen Publishing)

FRUITS AND VEGETABLES

Whenever possible, buy organically grown fruits and vegetables.

OLIVE OIL

Always buy extra virgin olive oil. Italy, Greece, and Spain all produce outstanding olive oils. Spanish olive oil is especially high in polyphenols.

ONLINE

For more information about Dr. Perricone, visit www.ThePerriconePrescription.com and iVillage.com's beauty site especially for women, Substance.com. Substance.com, the world's largest online beauty destination, has partnered with Dr. Perricone to give you personalized advice about his revolutionary prescription for staying young. At Substance.com you can: read excerpts from his #1 *New York Times* bestsellers, *The Perricone Prescription* and *The Wrinkle Cure*; get answers to his most frequently asked questions; sign up to receive a *free* newsletter from Dr. Perricone himself; and talk to other women about their successful experiences with the Perricone plan. You can also find the most up-to-date information on Dr. Perricone's television appearances, as well as a schedule for his live chats on Substance.com.

Visit www.iVillage.com/perricone
and
www.ThePerriconePrescription.com

For a more comprehensive list of recommended products and services, please see *The Perricone Prescription: A Physician's 28-Day Program for Total Body and Face Rejuvenation.*

Notes

Notes

Notes

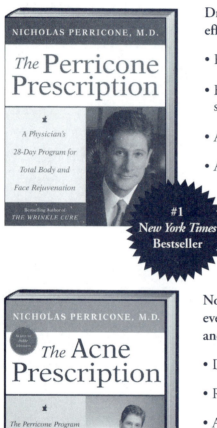